MAKING SENSE OF CLINICAL GOVERNANCE

A workbook for NHS doctors, nurses and managers

Roy Lilley

Foreword by

Richard Baker
*Director, Clinical Governance Research and Development Unit
University of Leicester*

RADCLIFFE MEDICAL PRESS

Radcliffe Medical Press Ltd
18 Marcham Road, Abingdon, Oxon OX14 1AA

British Library Cataloguing in Publication Data

A catalogue record for this book is available from the British Library.

ISBN 1 85775 425 5

Typeset by Advance Typesetting Ltd, Oxon.
Printed and bound by Hobbs the Printers, Totton, Hampshire.

CONTENTS

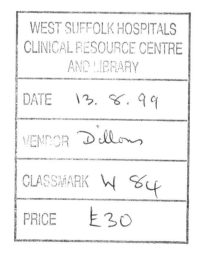

FOREWORD

Clinical governance is the new system for monitoring and improving quality in the NHS. Everyone has to be involved and as it evolves in the next few years, clinical governance will play an increasingly important part in our working lives. Therefore, we all need to learn more about it.

Yet at first sight, clinical governance can seem a difficult concept to grasp. It appears to be a confusing blend of many different activities and, if pressed, most health professionals would say that they have precious little time or energy to tackle any one of the activities in great depth. Also, many health professionals are anxious that clinical governance might imply greater control over their work. At the same time, managers are likely to be uncertain about methods of introducing clinical governance into their organisations. They will have concerns about the new system of accountability for the quality of care.

In fact, at the heart of clinical governance there is a very clear idea: it is doing anything and everything required to maximise quality. Roy Lilley makes this apparent in an approachable and understandable way. I enjoyed the workbook because it is practical but at the same time does not pretend that clinical governance is simpler or easier than it really is. It is fun to read but the content is enough to challenge anyone, and it would be difficult to use it without developing some new ideas.

I am pleased to recommend this book to you. Everyone involved in clinical governance will learn something from these pages, including nurses, doctors, medical and clinical directors, managers and staff supporting quality improvement activities in the health service. It will be equally valuable to those working in hospitals, the community or in primary care.

Richard Baker
Director, Clinical Governance Research and Development Unit
Department of General Practice and Primary Health Care
University of Leicester
May 1999

PREFACE

As someone with a background in industry, it is difficult for me to understand why the NHS makes such a fuss about quality. After all, quality is only about finding out what works and making sure you get it next time, the time after that and every time! What is more simple than getting people to do the job right, first time, every time? Ho, ho! If only it was that simple!

However, it is worth adding '… in the complex world of healthcare there cannot be any room for half measures, sloppy workmanship, or the waste of having to do things over again'. Who said that? Well, first exercise: find out!

In the caring and compassionate world of the NHS, where some people care about care more than caring itself, there is no room for rude people, insensitive people and people who cannot understand what it must be like not to understand. There cannot be any room for tests, treatments and procedures that don't work or are not done right – first time, every time.

It all sounds so easy, doesn't it? If only it was! The NHS has been rocked to its foundations by the inexplicable goings on at some of our greatest hospitals. The Service has been stunned by failures in screening and diagnostic services. How can it happen? No one sets out to blunder, no one wants to work in anything but a quality service. Well, the answer is easy. Quality is everybody's business and unless everybody is playing their part, quality soon disappears.

That's the trick. In industry we would look at quality as a continuum. Our task would be to manage the interfaces between services. In other words, join up the elements of the services we offer and make sure they are as good at the beginning as they are at the end.

Quality is like the red stripe in the toothpaste: no matter where you squeeze the tube and no matter how much there is left, the red stripe is always there.

Clinical governance (CG) is aiming to put the red stripe – the quality stripe – into the NHS.

CG is a term that many people find difficult to understand. The two words do seem unlikely partners. Think of it another way. Think of 'corporate governance'. You know, all that stuff about making sure the company's balance sheet adds up, that no one is on the fiddle, that procurement is carried out in an open and fair way, that remuneration is reasonable and rewarding. Things like Boards keeping a proper record of their decisions, paying suppliers on time, planning financial developments and staying within the company's overdraft limits. It is a simple concept, isn't it? Somehow you know instinctively what corporate governance means. Running the show properly!

Now think about CG in the same light. Suddenly it all becomes clear. CG is the total of all the factors that makes the NHS and the place where you work safe, using the best treatments there are, carried out by people who are up to date and know what they are doing. CG means having systems in place to spot when things are going wrong and being able to put them right, quickly and without a fuss. It also means having systems in place to spot good things and incorporate them into what you are doing, as fast as you can, every time.

CG means giving patients the reassurance that the NHS will do everything it can to get it right, first time, every time. And, when it doesn't, it will sort it out without making a fuss or turning the experience into a battle.

In any organisation there is no great sin in getting something wrong – it happens. The sin is not recognising it is wrong and doing something about it, making sure it doesn't go wrong again.

CG builds on the idea that quality is everyone's responsibility, we can all play our part. The patient's passage through an episode of sickness that takes them back to wellness involves scores of people. The car park attendant and the consultant surgeon, from the cleaner across to the community nurse, we all have a part to play. CG is about making sure everyone plays their part and gets it right, first time, every time. CG is about finding out what works best and doing our best to use it, in the best interest of our patients, residents, clients, carers, families and friends.

CG is long overdue and is a great opportunity for the NHS to prove it can do even better. It is not a mill stone but a stepping stone.

Enjoy the journey.

Roy Lilley
May 1999

> CG builds on the idea that quality is everyone's responsibility – we can all play our part. The patient's passage through an episode of sickness that takes them back to wellness involves scores of people. The car park attendant and the consultant surgeon, from the cleaner across to the community nurse, we all have a part to play.

ABOUT THE AUTHOR

Roy Lilley is a visiting fellow at the Management School, Imperial College London. He is a writer and broadcaster on health and social issues and has published nearly a dozen books on health and health service management and related topics.

As a former NHS Trust chairman, his Trust became the first to achieve BS 5750 (ISO 9001) quality accreditation for the whole of their services along with Investors in People approval for the whole of their HR and training strategies.

All staff took part in performance management and everyone had a personal development plan.

In 1991, the Trust established the 'QUIT' department. It stood for 'quitting bad habits', and involved a programme of total quality management that was recognised in industry but considered pioneering in the NHS. It went on to involve all staff and became the forerunner of a programme that today we would recognise as clinical governance.

Roy Lilley now works across the NHS to help with the challenges of modern management and is an enthusiast for radical policies that address the real needs of patients, professionals and the communities they serve.

By the same author:

- *The PCG Tool Kit*, second edition
- *The PCG Team Builder*, with Gareth Davies and Bill Cain
- *Writing Investment Plans and HImPs*
- *Making Sense of Risk Management*, with Paul Lambden

All published by Radcliffe Medical Press.

All the books in my PCG series have been dedicated to the army of NHS managers, clinicians and medical staff who have influenced my understanding of our greatest public service. I thanked them for the time they had taken and for sharing their insights, knowledge and experiences.

It would also be right to dedicate this book to my former colleagues at the now defunct Homewood NHS Trust in Surrey, where we learned that process control in quality is vital, but not as important as understanding what patients really want, and going out of your way to make sure they get it.

And, once again to A-T R, who brings the quality into my life.

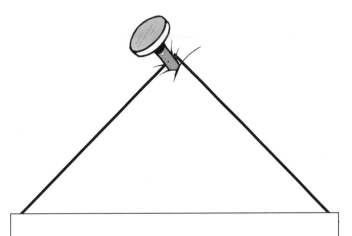

Quality is 'knowing what outcome you want and being sure you get it, every time, for as long as you want it.'

There are hundreds of definitions of what 'quality' is. This is the best one I can find. Oh all right, yes it's my definition, but it seems to me straightforward to understand and recognises that 'quality' is not just a process, it is an outcome and has its foundations in consistency. Plus, it can be changed, upgraded or dumped for something better. So, just in case there is any confusion, rip out this page and pin it on the notice board. Be sure you do because, one day, I might just come and visit your place and I'll be looking for it!

MAKING THIS WORKBOOK WORK FOR YOU

If you have seen any of the other workbooks in the PCG series, you will know the next bit off by heart. If you are new to the PCG workbook series, there is a bit of a shock coming!

There is no conventional beginning, middle or end to this book, so don't feel obliged to sit down and read it from cover to cover in a nice ordered way. Instead, flip through the pages and get a feel for what it has to offer. Not all of it will be of interest to you – skip those bits. Pick out the sections that look like they can help. This is a workbook, so make it work for you. Flip through the pages and make friends with it! Do it now and then come back to this page.

Welcome back!

I hope you have come across things in the book that you know already and, hopefully, some things you've never thought of. Perhaps even some stuff to make you think.

There are a number of **THINK BOXES** to get the juices flowing and to get you thinking outside the box and look at the issues from a different dimension. Some are deliberately provocative, some just for fun.

Hazard Warnings are there to point out some tricky issues, or traps not to fall into.

TIPS The **Tips** are short cuts and quick fixes to get you to the answer faster.

The **Exercises** are there for you to address the issues in the context of where you work and what your task is, regardless of your profession or seniority in the organisation. Use them to develop your own thinking or for brainstorming the issues with colleagues.

There are a lot of questions and no answers. This is not a 'right' or 'wrong' book: it asks the questions in the context of the issues in the hope that they will help you not to overlook an important topic or duck some of the tricky ones.

This is a non-threatening, environmentally friendly, non-genetically modified, unashamedly irreverently written, fun to play with book that tries to make CG easy.

Write on the pages, rip bits out, argue with it and throw it at the cat! Use it as a workbook to prove that not everything in life has to be serious to be good. Well, that's the idea. What do you think?

SECTION 1

Never mind the width,
what about the quality?

In case you have been protesting about a new bypass and living down a hole with Swampy, and you don't already know, here are the top line important things. In fact, the 'Dummy's Guide' to clinical governance. Rip it out and stick it on the fridge door with one of those funny magnet things, or stick it on the notice board in the office to make it look like you know what you're talking about.

- Processes are to be put in place to integrate quality into the organisation's processes. It's not a departmental issue anymore, now it's every-body's business.
- Quality is a lot about leadership and that leadership is to stem from clinical team level.
- Evidence-based practice, backed up by ideas and evaluated innovation will be systematically cascaded through the NHS.
- Clinical risk reduction programmes will be introduced.
- There will be a greater openness in detecting and investigating adverse events.
- Patients will be listened to and lessons learned from their experiences.
- Poor clinical performance will be detected earlier, to protect clinicians and patients.
- Clinical governance is the key theme in professional development.
- Improvements to the quality of clinical data captured.

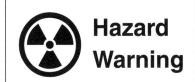 **Hazard Warning**

If someone wants to blow the whistle, how easy is it for your organisation to hear it?

How do you separate out the meddlesome from the well intended?

In short, the NHS is finding out what industry has known for years: quality is everybody's business.

OK, that's the basics – what else?

None of this is going to happen over night. There is a lot that is good in the NHS but a lot of it ain't so good. So, the idea of CG is that it is to be 'developmental'. This is the Department of Health's way of saying 'we know it's going to take time'. The Department of Health is also saying that although it knows it is going to take time, that's no excuse for not doing anything.

So, there are some benchmarks on the way.

One good thing (or perhaps not) is that the Department of Health is not being prescriptive. In other words, they are not defining the exact methods that are to be used but setting out a framework along with some key principles. The rest is up to you.

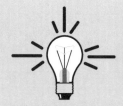

THINK BOX

If the NHS is serious about CG and quality, is it right to leave so much of the implementation up to the locals? Is this how Marks and Sparks do it? How can there be consistent quality in the NHS if everyone is being left to do their own thing? On the other hand, how much store is to be set against the ownership of a quality strategy? If folk don't own it, they won't do it and mean it.

So, in short, here are all the important bits, on one page:

Clinical governance is:

- everyone's business
- involving patients and service users
- ignoring departmental and service boundaries and works across them
- involving everyone in developing their professional capabilities
- continuous and evolving in its quest for improvement
- finding out what works best and doing it, every time
- based on evidence
- transparent and open.

Clinical governance is not:

- a stick to bash the doctors with
- another management fad
- a 'blame' thing
- tribal
- an excuse for not doing things
- up to someone else to do
- keeping quiet about things that go wrong.

Clinical governance recognises that:

A quality service is built by: being open about the strengths and weaknesses of what we do; being determined to improve by adopting and sharing the best practice we can find; making our own contribution more valuable through continuous personal development, comparing ourselves with the best; and by listening to the people we serve.

And here is what it 'looks' like …

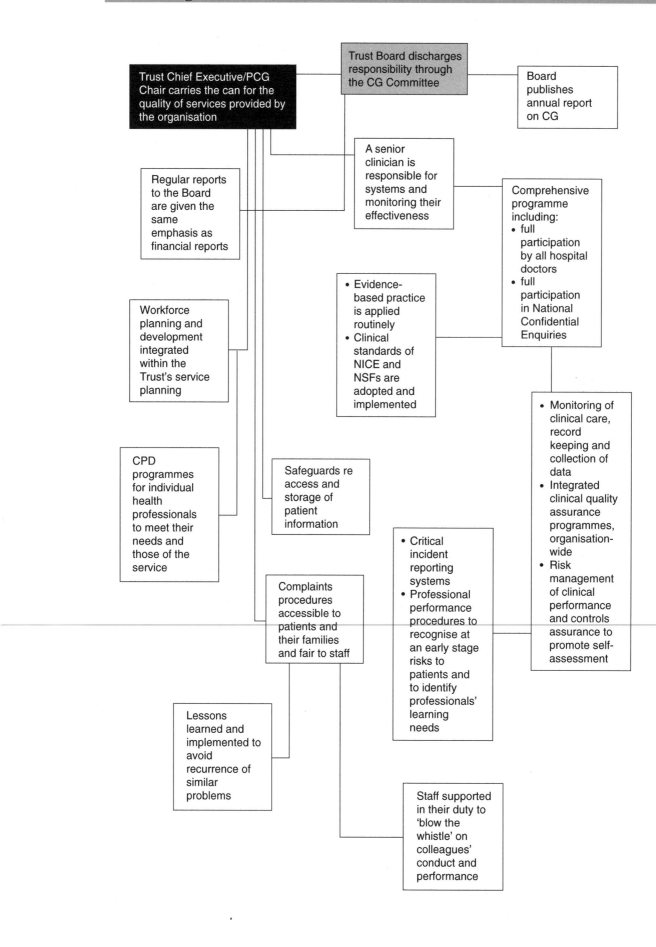

Trust Board discharges responsibility through the CG Committee

Trust Chief Executive/PCG Chair carries the can for the quality of services provided by the organisation

Board publishes annual report on CG

A senior clinician is responsible for systems and monitoring their effectiveness

Regular reports to the Board are given the same emphasis as financial reports

Comprehensive programme including:
• full participation by all hospital doctors
• full participation in National Confidential Enquiries

Workforce planning and development integrated within the Trust's service planning

• Evidence-based practice is applied routinely
• Clinical standards of NICE and NSFs are adopted and implemented

• Monitoring of clinical care, record keeping and collection of data
• Integrated clinical quality assurance programmes, organisation-wide
• Risk management of clinical performance and controls assurance to promote self-assessment

CPD programmes for individual health professionals to meet their needs and those of the service

Safeguards re access and storage of patient information

Complaints procedures accessible to patients and their families and fair to staff

• Critical incident reporting systems
• Professional performance procedures to recognise at an early stage risks to patients and to identify professionals' learning needs

Lessons learned and implemented to avoid recurrence of similar problems

Staff supported in their duty to 'blow the whistle' on colleagues' conduct and performance

If you haven't got around to it yet, now is a good time to make a cup of coffee and read the White Paper, *A First Class Service*.

You really should have read it by now, but I forgive you as you've got so much else on at the moment. So, I'll wait …

If you want to cheat, here are the five headline issues.

In short the aims are to:

1 tackle the causes of ill health
2 make services quick and easy to use
3 ensure the consistency of services, regardless of where you live
4 try and provide joined up services that are not constrained by artificial barriers between services, such as health and social services
5 spend money on equipment, buildings and staff.

Get the idea? Let's see…

Exercise

 Think about the aims in the five above headings and write down what part clinical governance could play in delivering them.

We are all going to get 10 years for this!

Relax, I don't mean we are going to jail. I mean that in the first White Paper, *The New NHS: modern, dependable*, they – whoever 'they' are – who wrote it … some say Sam Galbraith and Tony Blair did it over one weekend at Number 10. Very sad! They should have been shopping at Sainsburys or at an Oasis concert … anyway, I digress, they envisaged a 10-year programme of rolling improvement in the NHS.

What? You haven't read *modern, dependable*! Shame on you! I'll let you cheat just once more. It only said three main things about quality. Here they are:

1 clear national standards, delivered through National Service Frameworks and the National Institute of Clinical Excellence
2 local delivery of quality services, delivered through CG and a statutory duty of quality (maybe you will end up in jail after all!), supported by lifelong learning programmes and professional self-regulation
3 monitoring of services through the Commission for Health Improvement (the NHS regulatory body that I call 'Off-sick') and the NHS Performance Framework. Oh, I nearly forgot the patient and user experience survey (expected to report that the doctors and the nurses were 'luverley').

Joining all that together is the concept of CG. Or, in other words:

'A framework through which NHS organisations are accountable for continuously improving the quality of their services and safeguarding high standards of care, by creating an environment in which excellence in clinical care will flourish.'

That's right out of the CG guidance and I couldn't have put it better myself. So, I didn't! I copied it out. Well, why not? Most guidance is dire, that's why no one reads it. So, credit where it is due! The use of the word 'flourish' is almost romantic. It is certainly horticultural!

Let's take a closer look at some of the issues.

Move up the curve or go to jail…

In the language of management guru-speak there is a phrase. It is 'the quality curve'. What it means is that at one end of the scale you will find organisations that work at the leading edge of quality and are world class, while at the other end there are the basket cases. Generally, we discover organisations, whether they are health organisations or not, around the middle of the curve.

It looks a bit like this:

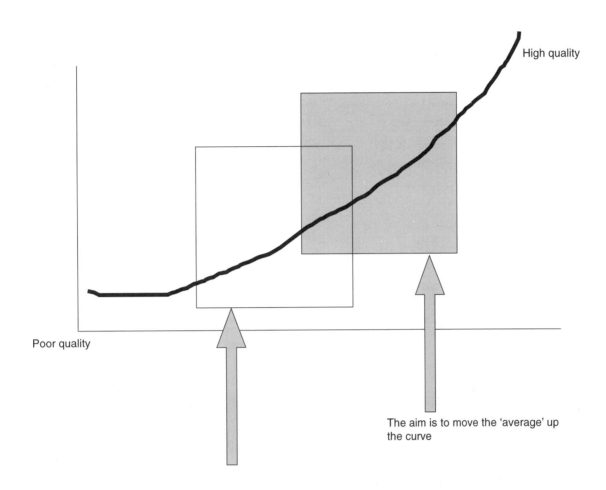

Part of the NHS's response, to get more of its units and organisations to move up the quality curve, is to introduce a concept called 'the statutory duty' of quality.

In other words: move up the curve or go to jail.

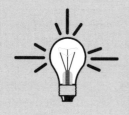

THINK BOX

What difference will threatening people with sanctions and punishment make to real quality in the NHS? Will the thought of appearing in the dock or being dragged before the Health Select Committee really make a district nurse, on her sixth visit of the day, in rainy, freezing cold, downtown Liverpool (sorry Liverpool) really make her do the job better? What does a statutory duty mean to you?

Learning from the best

The question I really want to ask is 'Who decides what's best?' You might want to think about that, too.

So do it ...

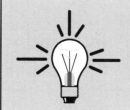

THINK BOX

Have a think. What really motivates people to do their jobs better? Threats, money, encouragement? What motivates you?

Anyway, there have been plenty of recent examples where anything but the best has emerged. The idea of CG is to cascade good practice into the NHS as fast as possible.

In effect, learning from leading edge outfits and getting them to pass on what they do. What does that mean for you and your organisation?

Exercise

 List the ways in which you personally (or your organisation) keep up to date with best practice.

What other things could you do?

Are there resource implications? What are they? Can you evaluate them? Can they be overcome?

Exercise

 Devise a way of evaluating your organisation's willingness to accept and adapt to change. Are people open and willing to having their present practice challenged?

Getting it together

With a bit of luck, by now you will have cottoned on to the idea that CG is about joining things together. Seeing quality in the round and understanding that it is everybody's business. Recognising the pathway through which a patient passes on their journey from sickness to wellness and making sure each part of that experience is flawless. As well as making sure that when we do things to and for folk, it is the best that we can do.

Exercise

 At the heart of delivering CG is getting people to be prepared to change what they do and work together. Can you evaluate your organisation's willingness to change? How would you make an evaluation so that you can go on to measure change when it takes place?

Exercise

How do you rate cross-departmental working at the moment? List the number of cross-functional teams that are presently working in your organisation and devise a system to look at their strengths and weaknesses.

We're OK, it's the others!

Where do you work? Primary care, secondary care, community care, on campus, off campus, special hospital, in a Trust? The truth is it doesn't matter. All this 'joined up ness' that the Department of Health is going on about will need a coherent strategy that will take the concept of CG into every part of the NHS. Mmm, now there's a thought.

Exercise

CG depends upon cross-service co-operation and joint working. Different services measure quality in different ways. How would you produce an audit model to evaluate a joint provided service?

How long have you got?

The Gods of Whitehall think this is a 10-year strategy. I wonder why. If it is so good and the NHS needs it so much, why take 10 years to do it. Can't it be done quicker than that?

Exercise

What are the reasons for taking 10 years over this? Can it be done quicker? Should it be done quicker? List the impediments to a speedier implementation of CG. How could they be overcome?

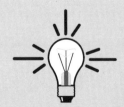

THINK BOX

Is the real reason it's going to take a decade to make it all happen, that it is about resources and we all know there ain't enough money in the NHS. How much of a part does money play in all this? Or is quality free?

CG is all about changing organisational culture and that means starting with you! No, perhaps not. You've been open-minded enough to get hold of a copy of this book and to stay with it this far! However, there is a nasty 'blame' culture in the NHS. It's tricky though. There is a fine line for managers and others to try and find.

The line between 'this person is a hopeless case, get rid of them' and 'this person has got it wrong, but with a bit of training and some help, they can do it better next time'.

Or 'it's their department, their fault and nothing to do with me'. Not easy, is it?

The hallmark of a good organisation is that it is open enough to recognise that from time to time things will go wrong and being willing to fix them.

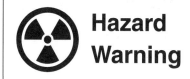

Hazard Warning

You can accuse someone of not being a very good driver. You might even suggest they are not the greatest lover in the world and live to tell the tale. But, when you start to challenge someone's clinical practice, look out! Be prepared for the roof to fall in!

Exercise

How's the 'culture' where you work? Does your place have a bad attitude? Can you define and measure the characteristics that are needed to move away from a 'blame' culture to an open culture and to become an organisation willing to learn from its mistakes and move on?

What happened? Did you see anything?

All this CG and other change stuff will have to be monitored. Otherwise, how will we know if we've done it!

Exercise

 Devise some foundation processes to start monitoring the improvement of quality in your organisation. They should not all be 'clinical' as the patient's journey may take them from the car park to the operating theatre and back again. And from the waiting room to the loo!

Too tough? Try this:

Exercise

 Will clinical governance bring any real benefits? List the benefits you would hope to see from a CG programme.

What about the vision thing?

We are starting to get an idea what it's all about, but what will it look like when it's finished? Does anyone have a vision?

If you like, describe the place you want to work in, in the following terms, then you'll have to share the vision thing. So, rip this page out and put it on your notice board or desk, or tape it on the wall.

Share the vision thing!

I want to work in a place that ...

1 is open and where education, research and sharing good practice are part of the everyday experience

2 makes quality everybody's business

3 routinely asks the customers what they want

   Yes, I mean customers because patients, relatives, carers, family and friends have in some way contributed to the taxes that pay for the NHS (and my wages and yours).

4 the Board and the bosses take as much notice of quality issues as they do finance

5 has good, up-to-date information that it can use to measure our progress and plan for the future.

   If you agree with me, shout hooray!
   And then, tell me what can we do about it?

Exercise

Carers play an important role in delivering quality care. This is a sensitive area. Sometimes, even well intentioned carers can get it very wrong. What action could you take to improve the knowledge, skills and attitudes of carers as part of a quality initiative?

Exercise

 Someone senior should be overseeing user, carer and public involvement strategy. Who is going to do it? How should the person be chosen and what are their key deliverables?

Exercise

 Is it a good idea to have a user representative on the clinical governance committee?

List the advantages and the disadvantages.

Exercise

 If it is a good idea to have a user representative on the clinical governance committee, how will the person be chosen?

How will you prevent them being single tracked on one disease area? How will you avoid them being too generalist?

How will you avoid the appointment being mere tokenism?

Exercise

 Describe what a training and induction programme for such a representative might look like.

What are the key issues they must understand?

Exercise

 Describe the role that focus groups and patient organisations might play.

How would you recruit people to take part?

Exercise

 What evidence is there that departments and individuals are currently sharing knowledge and good practice? For example, when a colleague attends a conference, do they routinely feed back to their department or group?

Exercise

 Are you reinventing the wheel?

Devise a strategy to ensure knowledge is shared.

Identify how you would establish what best practice is, in any given area or speciality.

Can you identify how much duplication of effort there is? How many people or departments are really trying to reinvent the wheel?

Exercise

Looking to improve clinical performance and securing better quality outcomes for patients? How would you deal with issues of poor individual practice?

Exercise

 Often, poor performing organisations will have started higher up the quality curve (remember that?) and for reasons of familiarity and poor management they slip. What are some other factors that contribute to slippage?

Devise a programme that will identify quality slippage and move the organisation towards a culture of sustained improvement.

SECTION 2

Let's get down to the nitty gritty

How's all this fine vision stuff going to be translated into things we can do, measure and get on with?

Well, it's not a bad question. The whole CG issue does start to have a bit of a touchy-feely air about it. The answer is: it is not supposed to be touchy-feely at all but systematic, sensible, practical and local. Everybody working together and all that jazz.

We know that it is about joined up services, so let's make a start with some integrated planning for quality care.

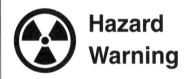 **Hazard Warning**

At the heart of all this is the intention to address deficiencies in services.

Toes are going to be trod upon and a few egos sent home in tears. This is not an easy ride. Some poor practice is so ingrained you'll have to get a JCB to dig it up.

Integrated planning

Think about the journey of a patient from wellness to sickness. One day they're fit as a flea, the next they are run over, have a heart attack or fall off a ladder. For others the experience of sickness will start as a slow loss of function that manifests itself as nothing more than a minor discomfort. Then, before you know it they are in big trouble. Whatever accident, illness or disease the patient experiences, the business of returning to function, or in the case of long-term care such as learning disability achieving optimal function, is not the product of one department, surgery, hospital or tertiary referral. A whole host of people are involved.

Getting colleagues to think vertically about their department is easy.

They can talk all day (and some do!) about how they can improve the patient experience for people who are looked after in their department. Getting them to think horizontally outside the box (outside their department) is a different issue. They only see the bit they do.

Unfortunately, most large organisations are arranged in vertical departments. Staff who work in this department or that only think about their bit.

Some businesses can get away with it. The good ones don't even try – they recognise the problem and deal with it.

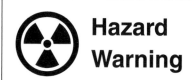 **Hazard Warning**

They can talk all day (and some do!) about how they can improve the patient experience for people who are looked after in their department. Getting them to think horizontally outside the box (outside their department) is a different issue. They only see the bit they do.

The NHS is the biggest remaining nationalised industry in the world. It is complex and divided vertically.

Customers travel 'across' from one department to the next, experiencing a range of elements in the total experience.

In the NHS the patient sees the whole picture and experiences the whole experience: good and bad. The idea is to start thinking about issues horizontally, not vertically.

Exercise

 Pick a disease area and look at it horizontally from the patient's perspective. From the first hint of a symptom to return to function. How many departments are involved? How many services? How many interfaces? Count them.

If you are stuck for an idea, try looking at the journey of an elderly patient needing a hip replacement.

No one plans to fail, they just fail to plan

Like all good things CG, if it works, will be the product of good planning. The plan has to start by identifying weaknesses in the services and trying to address them in the Health Improvement Programme (HImP).

What are HImPs?

Shame on you! Have you been away attempting a long-distance balloon record or something?

Here's a quick over view:

HImPs are the new planning tool designed to bring together health authorities, local government, PCGs, Trusts and a host of stakeholders to identify the health needs of an area. In other words, take a horizontal look at the services.

If you want to know more about HImPs, there is a great book on the subject published by Radcliffe Medical Press. Modesty forbids me from identifying the author!

They are also a good place to start to identify parts of the service that might be in need of a makeover. It is likely that quality issues will identify themselves during the HImP needs assessment phase:

• quality issues may well emerge because other agencies will be looking at the services, coming at the issues with a fresh pair of eyes

and

• quality issues identified and addressed in a HImP are likely to have a much wider applicability for other local services. You see, it's all this 'joined-upness' again.

So use the HImP as an opportunity to identify quality issues and address them across the boundaries of care.

Exercise

 Identify an illness or disease area (perhaps dementia), that impacts across a number of services: housing, health, social services, voluntary sector. How do you make quality central to joint working?

What about the workers?

If you want to talk quality, you've got to talk people. You can have all the systems, processes and checks you want but in the end organisations depend on people.

What are your people like?

In the 'guru speak' of the management consultant we need to do a bit of 'workforce planning'. Sounds boring? No, you're wrong. This is 'acetastin'superfizzin'lip-smackin'excitin' stuff.

Mind the gap

The trick here is to try and close the gap between what the services are like now and what you want them to be. Then take a stab at what that means for staff, the number employed, their competencies and their training.

For example, if your PCG decides it wants to deliver more services through a health visitor network, the question is: how many health visitors do you need, how many have you got now and what extra skills will they need to deliver this super new service?

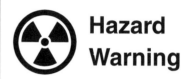

Hazard Warning

For reasons of demography, age, skill mix, rewards and working conditions, in some parts of the UK nurses are becoming as rare as mermaids.

This all gets a lot more difficult when you start to talk about nursing. For reasons of demography, age, skill mix, rewards and working conditions, in some parts of the UK nurses are becoming as rare as mermaids. Indeed, the Gods of Whitehall are so worried about it that there are all sorts of initiatives under way to try and encourage newcomers into the profession, and to stem the flow of nurses leaving the NHS. The problem is they can often get a better deal working for a pharma company or Marks and Sparks. And, on top of that, to get some of the nurses that have left the NHS to come back. None of this is easy and all of it takes time – probably longer than you've got! So beware …

The situation with GPs is not much better. About one-third of vacancies on vocational courses to become GPs are empty. Getting GPs to work in some inner city settings is very tough indeed. So, don't underestimate how tough the general workforce planning issues can be.

Exercise

 Consider the workforce planning issues where you work. What members of staff or professions do you have most trouble recruiting and retaining? What actions can you take to change the situation?

What services might be in jeopardy if workforce planning issues aren't addressed?

Are workforce planning issues preventing you from offering new services? What can you do to address the problem?

How good is the team?

Exercise

 Devise a method of auditing the current skills of the workforce available to you. Don't assume everyone at the same grade will have the same skills. You must include a way of establishing an up-to-date record of how they have 'up skilled' themselves (by going on courses etc) that you may not be aware of. What special interests have they acquired that are useful to the organisation?

Exercise

 Is there a need to develop a new group, or team, of staff with a set of skills and competencies that will help deliver CG?

Explain how you would assess the need for new skills and competencies and how you would go about establishing the development needs of the group.

Help is at hand

If all this workforce 'thingamajig' is new to you, don't worry. Everyone else is just as confused!

Here is a list of folk who will probably be able to lend you a hand and point you in the right direction, giving you some ideas. Now is the time to go and be nice to lots of new people – oh, what fun!

- Regional education and development groups
- Education and training consortia
- Postgraduate deans
- Local medical workforce advisory groups.

And, don't forget the director of human resources at the Trust hospital. They will know a thing or two about all this – and it's about time we gave them something useful to do! But don't tell 'em I said so!

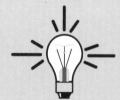

THINK BOX

Continuing professional development (CPD) is something of a mystery. Doctors get points for going to meetings, many of which are sponsored by pharma companies, that turn out to be not much more than a bit of a jolly. Can you partner a pharma company to do something really useful around CPD and CG? Most of the pharma companies are gagging to get on board the PCG train and many of them have a genuine desire to get a better understanding of CG. Are there ethical reasons that prevent a closer working relationship with a pharma company, or is a well-defined and sensible relationship something to work for? Does your organisation have a policy about such matters? If not, why not?

There is another group of folk you can turn to for some help. Go and see them. More meetings!

- Clinical tutors

- Royal College tutors

- Regional directors of education and training.

Exercise

 The NHS has a whole network of library services that can be used to support CG.

Devise and carry out an audit of library services and design a programme to develop linkages with the various reference and library resources to make the pool of knowledge accessible and available.

Consider the role of IT in the process.

Time for a cup of coffee and to read the NHS Human Resource Strategy Document, *The New NHS: working together, securing a quality workforce for the NHS*. Who thinks up these titles? Heaven help us (or them). Stuck for a copy? Try the HR department of a Trust or download a copy from the Department of Health website. What, not wired? No access to the Internet? Consider early retirement.

Exercise

Set in the context of CG, what are the training and education needs of the organisation? Devise a method of matching the organisational requirements around CG and the skills needed by the staff to deliver the agenda. Tough job? Yes it is. But, there is no point trying to deliver an organisational agenda without knowing whether or not the troops can deliver it. So, tough exercise yes, but a tougher world without it.

You can have a second coffee, or something stronger, whilst you figure this one out!

Exercise

Each employee should have a training and development plan. How would you assess the training needs of the individual? Do they have to be job related or can the development be 'personal development'?

Exercise

What benchmarks can you establish and put in place to ensure the individual is benefiting from development training?

Can anybody tell me what's going on?

In so far as CG can be seen as a quality improvement programme, good information is vital.

Exercise

How would you use an information strategy to assess the scope for improvement within available resources?

Exercise

What information would be required to ensure that a quality improvement plan or investment has delivered the changes you want? How would you monitor progress to prevent slippage and how would you compare outcome against ambition?

Exercise

Where similar services are available elsewhere, how would you develop a system to benchmark your progress against others and identify scope for improvement? Start by taking one service, say asthma clinics for adults or fracture clinics, and devise a benchmarking formula.

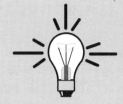

THINK BOX

With a view to openness and accountability, how would you inform the public about the quality of services provided by your organisation? Would you be prepared to highlight poor services? Should you? Is it as important to tell the public about the bad things as it is the good things? Should they know? Would it inform them or frighten them?

Exercise

Consider the impact of some recent NHS failings on public confidence in the Service. Do people really get frightened or do they just imagine 'it won't happen to them'?

In truth they have very little choice but to trust their local services. Explain how you would rejuvenate public confidence in women's screening programmes.

In the best of well run organisations, things can go wrong. What happens then? The NHS has had more than its fair share of blunders and foul ups. CG is about trying to prevent them happening. Information is vital to the process.

Exercise

With the aim of getting an early warning of serious service failures, devise a system to monitor outcomes of care that can spot trends. How would you present this information to the Board, many of whom will be unfamiliar with the detail of clinical issues?

Hazard Warning

Most NHS information systems are nowhere near as good as the type of information systems that are available to industry. We have a long way to go. The new IT strategy will improve things over time. Not read it yet? Shame on you, particularly if you are working in primary care. Most of the changes and improvements start in your backyard. So beware of the information that is currently available in the NHS. Much of it is old and a lot of it is not very accurate. Placing too great a reliance on it can lead to wrong assumptions, poor decisions and a future flipping hamburgers.

Exercise

 Devise some small-scale initiatives within a particular service to demonstrate the quality of what is being provided. Take into account clinical and non-clinical issues.

Exercise

 In the broader context of CG what type of information should be routinely gathered? Take into account comparisons with national data and both clinical and non-clinical data.

Still not read the IM&T strategy? I'm starting to wonder about your bedside reading. OK, here's the 'Bluffers Guide'. I wouldn't want any friend of mine to be unable to bluff their way around the IT strategy! It is important because a lot of CG strategy depends on information. So, if you can't 'do' technology, think of a career in tattooing or something useful.

- The much criticised IMG is scrapped and replaced by the NHS Information Authority (NHSIA): a special health authority dealing with strategy and integrating IT into the NHS 'family'.
- A 'sharply focused' Information Policy Unit will be set up in the NHSE.
- Establish electronic patient records (EPR) for every patient in the country, starting in PCGs with 'more detailed' records later in the acute sector.
- 24-hour access online to EPR **and** information on best clinical practice.
- 'Seamless care' through primary, secondary and community care.
- Public online access to health information.
- More care through telemedicine and NHS Direct.
- Provide health planners with data for resource management.
- Widespread consultation with public and professional groups to establish a **new** national body for security of personal health information.
- Appoint local 'guardians of patient privacy' (implemented by April 1999).
- By the end of 1999 all GP practices to be able to communicate with hospitals for test results.
- By 2002 all GP practices to be able to book hospital appointments electronically and exchange information about referrals, discharge and results.
- By 2002 implementation of Beacon electronic health records sites.
- A Clinical Information Management Programme **and** Clinical Data Standards Board to develop national clinical data standards for clinical terms, coding and classification.
- A register to provide an umbrella for:
  - new electronic health records
  - clinical electronic data interchange
  - decision support
  - stock control
  - costing adverse drug reaction reporting
  - performance management
  - care delivery systems.
- National Electronic Library for Health – another new organisation for:
  - harnessing health information on the worldwide web
  - supporting bedside and desktop clinical decisions
  - a closed network with access extended to patients and the general public as well as clinicians and managers
  - 'leading edge' decision support for clinicians which is centrally funded, evaluated and accredited.

You want it when!

Here's the timescale for IM&T implementation:

1 ensure millennium issues
2 develop costed local implementation strategies
3 completion of essential infrastructure
4 connect all GPs to the NHSNet
5 widen NHS Direct as a national service
6 complete NHS e-mail connections
7 establish local health information services
8 complete cancer information strategy
9 Beacon EHR sites completed
10 35% of acute hospitals to have EPR, integrated patient master index, patient administration, departmental systems, electronic clinical orders, results reporting, prescribing and multi-professional care pathways
11 25% of health authorities to have EPRs
12 NHSNet used for bookings, referrals, radiology, lab requests/results, nationwide
13 GP prescribing, electronic links to pharmacy and the Prescription Prescribing Authority
14 Telemedicine options routinely considered
15 National Library for Health accessible through local intranets
16 Information strategies underpinning national service frameworks
17 Beacon HER sites operational.

1999

2002

Exercise

 Drawing on the outcome of the previous exercise, identify how you would develop an information technology infrastructure to support CG. What are the key components?

Exercise

The recurring theme throughout government policy is for all the agencies involved in health, in its broadest possible definition, to work together as partners. The 'joined-up' thing. Sharing information is a start.

Design a method of auditing the IT status of your existing partners, to establish duplication and overlap and then consider what policies you would have to put in place to ensure all agencies work together. Take into account social services, the voluntary sector and all agencies that are likely to contribute to a HImP.

Consider common IT platforms, skills levels and training needs.

Are we marching in step?

Gathering this information is all very well but what does it mean? You could be marching along thinking everything is beautiful, the sun is shining, God is in his (or her) heaven and all is right with the world. And then, some hairy NCO taps you on the shoulder and tells you that everyone else turned left three miles ago. Oops!

There is no point in finding out how you are doing if you don't have systems to find out how everyone else is doing and comparing your performance with the rest. You never know, you might be the best ... Well, stranger things have happened!

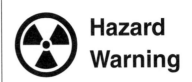

Hazard Warning

It won't be long before variations in performance will be more transparent than they have ever been in the history of the NHS.

With the aim of stringing together good practice and to get everyone working in the same way, the Gods of Whitehall have come up with the bright idea of NHS Performance Assessment Frameworks and an associated set of High Level Performance Indicators (HLPIs) to provide comparative information on performance, relative to similar organisations.

Good, eh?

In short, this means there will be a common set of data that you will be expected to provide – some 'grey suit', working in a dungeon in Leeds, will then number crunch everything and publish a set of results, so you can see how you are doing. You'll be compared against the norm – 'good old Norm', always was a bit of a laugh.

The set of HLPIs will include a set of clinical indicators that will be published sometime in the future. No doubt, just as soon as the grey suits can agree with the white coats.

It is probably safe to assume that the first stab at it will include the old chestnuts of mortality and readmission rates following heart attack and hip replacement, on a hospital by hospital basis.

And, no doubt more will follow.

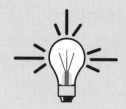

THINK BOX

The BMA and other doctors' groups have traditionally been against publishing outcome data. One of their leaders Jim Johnson once famously, and I think insultingly, said that the public would not be able to understand it and it would frighten them.

Well, now it's all change with the docs. They seem to have dropped their opposition, at least for the time being. That is not to say a punch-up may not occur in the future but, for now, they are ominously quiet. Probably something to do with the tragic events at a certain hospital and a string of foul-ups in screening departments. There wasn't much they could say about all that.

Are Jim and his mates right? Will the public understand it? For example, about 9% of hip replacements have to be done again, sometimes with very good reason. Such things as case mix, the age of the patient, their general state of health, whether the tissue shrinks around the prosthesis and so on.

So if a hospital has a higher than 9% average of what the docs euphemistically call 'revision rate', does it really mean a bad hospital and rubbish docs?

No, it doesn't. But great care will have to be taken to ensure the information is presented in a way the public will find useful and informative and doesn't frighten them off. **Perhaps Jim was right all along!**

What do you think?

Exercise

 Describe how you would present complex, case mix weighted, patient status information, outcome data to the public, in a way that would be helpful to them.

Different strokes for different folks

It is clear that information is one thing, but presenting it for different audiences and different consumption is quite another.

If this is all starting to look like evidence-based clinical decision making, you are right!

Health professionals making clinical decisions will require a different diet of data. When you think of the number of clinicians there are in the NHS and the potential for variations in their approach to treatment, you can appreciate that good dissemination of information is vital. How to do it is the problem. Doctors have traditionally not been too keen on the idea of being told what to do. They are very bright boys and girls and if you are going to try and change their practice, you can only do it on the basis of the evidence and you have to be pretty darned sure the evidence is real good!

Gathering information and tailoring it to the needs of the health professional, supporting the clinical decisions they are making, means focusing on how the evidence is made available to them.

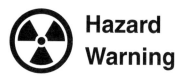 **Hazard Warning**

Doctors have traditionally not been too keen on the idea of being told what to do. They are very bright boys and girls and if you are going to try and change their practice, you can only do it on the basis of the evidence and you have to be pretty darned sure the evidence is real good!

Presenting the evidence and making it accessible is vital. At the moment, information systems (not just electronic ones) resemble the Tower of Babel, on a bad day.

The aim of CG is to bring some uniformity to the presentation of the evidence, to ensure it is up-to-date, convenient and properly research based.

How to do it? There's a good question!

Here is a list of some of the existing sources of good information:

The Cochrane Library

This is made up of four databases:

- Cochrane Database of Systematic Reviews
- Database of Abstracts of Reviews of Effectiveness
- Cochrane Controlled Trials Register
- Cochrane Reviews Methodology Database.

 A visit to their website is strongly recommended as a good use of lunchtime. What, not wired? Go and cut the lawn with a pair of nail clippers …

The NHS Centre for Review and Dissemination (CRD)

If you have ever wondered where *Effective Health Care Bulletins* and *Effectiveness Matters* come from, this is the place. The CRD commissions and supports reviewers to undertake reviews on areas of importance and produces summaries of research evidence. They are topic based.

The National Research Register

These good folk provide information on research that is already underway in the NHS. The idea being to stop other people trying to re-invent the wheel.

Wait, there is more …

The National Institute for Clinical Excellence (NICE)

You must have overdosed on cough medicine and be fast asleep if you haven't come across this lot. It is a special health authority, appointed by the Secretary of State, to establish and promote clinical and cost effectiveness. Note the reference to 'cost'. To some, this looks like the Department of Rationing. Once it gets going it will churn out 'high quality, evidenced-based' guidelines for the management of diseases and the use of significant new and existing interventions. So, now you know.

Hazard Warning

NICE is very likely to produce a row with the pharmaceutical industry who may find it more difficult to introduce expensive therapies into the NHS – **and** a moral and ethical punch-up between NICE and doctors who want to prescribe something that NICE thinks is too expensive. Look out for a challenge in the European Courts. Some say NICE is outside EC Health Directive 105 1989.

What, you don't know about it? Well you'll just have to go and find out because there is no room to start a discussion about Europe here!

The National Electronic Library for Health

Sounds familiar? Well, it should. It is part of the NHS Information Strategy – see the 'Bluffers Guide' on p. 49. It plans to include 'loadsagoodstuff' including summaries of primary and secondary research evidence, systematic reviews and evidence-based guidance to support clinical decision making and learning.

Exercise

 There's a lot of information about. Devise a way to monitor professional staff's access to the information that ensures the practice is up-to-date and improving the quality of what they do.

Exercise

Describe how you would deal with a clinician who resists accessing knowledge that might improve their practice. Consider barriers that are technology based. Is the clinician unhappy with IT-based systems? What is the role of peer pressure? Does the clinician mistrust the evidence? What other factors may come into play? Describe how you would identify and deal with them.

Exercise

 Develop a local infrastructure to inform the process of CG, to cascade best practice, improve practice and educate the clinical process. Consider bulletins, newsletters and computer-based systems. Consider the amount of information already in the system and how your approach would command attention and be more convenient.

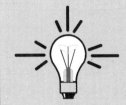

THINK BOX

There's a lot of it about. Information I mean. If I were a doctor, I don't know where I'd begin in trying to keep up-to-date and still have enough time to see patients. In the guidance issued by the Department of Health there are five sources of information that will form the basis of familiarising clinical performance and improving practice. Five! On top of that there are hundreds of magazines, circulars, newsletters, websites and goodness knows what else, in hundreds of different formats. Local groups are also being encouraged to have their own information infrastructure as part of their CG planning. Is it likely that the five sources of information featured by the DoH itself will be too much? Doesn't the real solution lie in a single entry point for information all presented in the same format? Can you ever have too much information?

What happens when it all goes wrong?

The tabloids love it and TV fills its news and current affairs programmes with special enthusiasm when the NHS gets it wrong. Banner headlines are the reward for a service that looks after millions of folk every year and gets just a handful of things wrong. Sometimes it seems like there isn't much justice. The trouble is, the NHS getting it wrong might be a one in a million mishap, but it is a personal tragedy for someone and their family and friends.

No one sets out in medicine to be a bad doctor or a sloppy nurse. None of the professionals working in healthcare wants to do anything but their best. However, we know don't we, that some clinicians and medics are better than others.

Poor performance is the scourge of the NHS and in an organisation that employs so many people it is often impossible to detect, until it is too late. Fortunately, foul-ups are rare and the vast majority of practitioners have high professional standards. But one mess-up has a disproportionate effect on the rest and has an impact on the public's confidence in the NHS.

Traditionally, the professions have been responsible for regulating themselves. That is likely to change and look out for developments about the future of self-regulation.

Recent experience has shown that self-regulation cannot be relied upon to provide the standards and reassurance the public is entitled to.

Some say the days of self-regulation are numbered. Credentialing and retraining and methods similar to those used by airlines for their pilots and other staff, are on the cards. This might mean a system emerging where, for a doctor to remain on the General Register, he or she would have to undergo re-accreditation every five years.

The performance of practitioners is closely aligned to CG. Professional self-regulation and CG sit side by side. The real responsibility lies at local level, close to where the practice is.

Procedures for all professional groups aimed at identifying and remedying poor performance, should include:

- critical incidents reporting to ensure that adverse events are identified, openly investigated, lessons are learnt and promptly applied
- complaints procedures which are accessible to patients and their families and are fair to staff
- disciplinary procedures which take effect at an early stage before patients are harmed and which help the individual to improve their performance whenever possible, in place and understood by all staff.

Exercise

 Looking to improve clinical performance and securing better quality outcomes for patients, describe how you would deal with issues of poor practice.

Exercise

Evaluate the complaint procedures where you work. Do they work swiftly? Do they produce results for patients? How would you assess the attitude of clinical colleagues to complaints from the public about their practice?

Do you think the process can be improved or speeded up? There are issues about liability and the prospect of legal action. Do they get in the way of good patient relations?

Did we learn anything?

In the best of well run organisations, from time to time things will go wrong. It is no sin. The sin is knowing that things are going wrong but doing nothing about putting them right, not learning and not ensuring that whatever it was cannot happen again.

CG is often portrayed in a policing role and in truth, in some senses, it is. But it is also about learning. It is about teaching as much as it is about policing. The Gods of Whitehall have woken up to the fact that the NHS has not always been so good about learning from adverse incidents and evaluating complaints. So the Chief Medical Officer (head honcho) and friends are having a look at how the NHS can learn from its mistakes. Yes, I know there's a lot to learn but at least they're making a start.

Watch this space.

Exercise

Evaluate how complaints are collected and analysed in your organisation. Develop a system to use them in a CG setting as part of learning and changing practice.

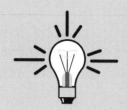

THINK BOX

What's wrong with professional self-regulation? Medicine is a complex business and who better than a medic to figure out if a medic is up to scratch or not? This is the argument used by the police service. Only a policeman can investigate a policeman because only a policeman is smart enough to catch a policeman.

Sounds like rubbish or sense? What are the alternatives for the NHS? Do we end up with a body similar to the Police Complaints Authority?

Is the real issue the relationships professionals, particularly doctors, have with one another? Careers can be made or ruined by senior consultants in their evaluation of junior colleagues. What junior doctor is going to risk being branded a trouble maker and blow the whistle on a senior colleague?

If it's good enough for you, it's good enough for me

The bit that's easy to forget about the health service is the 'national' bit. We are all focused on where we work and it is easy to overlook the fact that up and down the country there will be 'loadsafolk' all doing the same thing. Some of what you are doing will be better than they are doing and some of what they are doing will be better than you. With close on a million people working in and for the NHS, there is bound to be duplication.

What does that mean for the people we serve? The residents, patients, clients and their relatives, carers and friends? It means that if someone doing your job in another part of the country has discovered a way to do it better, then the folk you are responsible for are not getting the best possible deal. Is that what you want? No, of course not.

The history of the NHS has been built on locally inspired innovations. The trick for the future is to find a way to cascade new ideas and best practice into the NHS as a whole. A systematic way to adopt the best of the best and to dump the rest.

Exercise

How would you set up a system to provide service-specific access to good practice? What other agencies and groups would you involve? How would you measure use and access? Consider the exercise in the context of where you work and then roll the answers into a national setting. How might the two approaches vary?

Treading on toes

Highlighting good practice means putting a spotlight into the dark corners of poor practice – something the NHS has, traditionally, been reluctant to do. Egos are fragile and toes are tender when trod upon. Reputations can be ruined or made. This is no easy task. The best way to highlight poor practice is to prompt practitioners to do it for themselves and to compare their approaches, practice and achievements with others working in the same type of service elsewhere.

Exercise

 What are the impediments preventing professionals examining and measuring their own performance against the performance of others? List them and consider ways of removing the difficulties. Do you consider this a clinical issue only? Should it be exclusively a clinical issue? Can managers and other non-medical colleagues be measured in the same way?

Is it really good?

What constitutes good practice? You may be convinced that the way you do it is the best way and everyone else is wrong. How do you know? The foundation of best practice is in the evidence.

Exercise

What are the factors that constitute good practice? How would you define evidence-based, good practice? Is it always possible to define it? What are the elements you would have to put in place to ensure that alleged good practice is actually evidence based?

Everybody's doing it

Gathering evidence about good practice is getting easier. Everybody is doing it. Many NHS organisations have worked with outside organisations or established their own networks. The British Association of Medical Managers has been in the forefront and the King's Fund has invented a commercial arm to their activities and moved into the shark-infested waters of quality assurance accreditation.

Other local initiatives have included:

• benchmarking clubs
• twinning
• exchange visits
• master classes.

I detect a genuine enthusiasm and interest in leveraging up quality and practice. There is no doubt that national initiatives have provided the impetus but real quality has to be owned and understood locally. The danger is that as the NHS strives to make good practice part of its culture, the effort becomes fragmented and the wheel reinvented a thousand times a day.

Technology should provide us with an answer. An NHS website was launched in March and can be found at:

www.doh.nhsweb.NHS.uk/NHS/clingov.htm

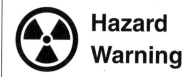

Hazard Warning

The danger is that as the NHS strives to make good practice part of its culture, the effort becomes fragmented and the wheel reinvented a thousand times a day.

Note that this is a national NHS website and cannot be accessed from outside.

The idea is that local services and interested staff can get in touch with each other to share good ideas and have a network on quality and CG issues. Remember, talking to colleagues in the firm's time is called networking, in your own time it is called gossip!

Off your trolley

There's 'loadsagoodstuff' on the NHSWeb. It will have a database of SDP – that's Whitehall speak for 'Service Delivery and Practice'. It means you will be able to enter details of all the good things you are doing to implement CG, plus all the other stuff you have to do about emergency admissions and making sure granny doesn't end up on a trolley in a corridor. And such things as managing waiting lists. The NHSWeb will be a fund of good ideas.

If you can't get on the web and don't do the IT stuff, you are going to have to have a serious word with someone. Your workplace should be on the Internet and if it isn't the propeller heads in the IT department should be able to tell you when you can expect to be hooked up. You remember the IT strategy thing? Well, they are supposed to be delivering it. So ring them up and pester them.

It is probably worthwhile investing in a piece of kit to use at home. PC Internet access is getting cheaper all the time and there's a whole world of learning and knowledge out there.

 If you are not wired, sit down with a cup of coffee and work out how you can get yourself hooked up. You are missing serious stuff.

For example, the NHS has a Learning Zone (nothing to do with the Dome) which is intended to carry an NHS Trust benchmarking database. Expect to see high level indicators of performance by Trusts added to the site. You'll then be able to compare what you are doing with the best of them.

Other topics will include:

- waiting lists and times (The Gods of Whitehall's Holy Grail)
- primary care issues
- mental health
- cancer services
- health improvement
- staff development.

And… information about Beacon services.

What are they? Beacon services are services within the NHS which have been selected as a particularly good example of what it does. More importantly, they will be given a few quid to disseminate learning to other NHS organisations and tell them about the good stuff they are doing.

This is a great idea. Beacon services are real NHS services who will have something to show you. They are not some wacky idea that an egg head has written about in a journal or picked up from the health service in Outer Mongolia. These are real services, run by real people, doing really good things.

People just like you who are struggling with the same problems and the same resource limitations. It'll be worth getting on the Net just for that alone.

And you can always do something good yourself, and become a Beacon outfit! Why not?

These are real services, run by real people, doing really good things. People just like you who are struggling with the same problems and the same resource limitations. It'll be worth getting on the Net just for that alone.

Exercise

Think about the services that are offered where you work. What is there that you are most proud of? Is there a service that really stands out as being good? What would you have to do to turn it into a Beacon service?

It's not just about flowers and clean loos

CG is about everything that impacts on the patient experience, plus a few things that you might not have considered.

In the past couple of years the NHS has implemented a 'controls assurance' policy. I bet you didn't know that! If you did, the chances are you are a senior manager or a finance type person. Controls assurance is about organisational risk management. That means having sound financial systems in place and parallel arrangements for assessing and managing non-financial and non-clinical risks. Things like the health and safety of staff and patients.

So, what do you do? Easy...

- Assess the likely level of risk.
- Decide where the risk is best managed.
- (For PCGs) create risk reserves and devise procedures for monitoring budgets through the year, decide when to release the reserves and agree how many calls on risk reserves will effect the following year's budget.

Exercise

 Make a list of potential risks and indicate where you think the risk should be managed.

SECTION 3

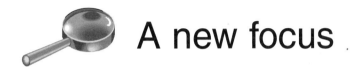 A new focus

Doing it horizontally

If clinical governance is anything it is the product of looking at services horizontally – joined up services – and recognising that a broken leg ends up fixed only after it has experienced perhaps:

- ambulance services
- waiting rooms
- triage
- examination
- X-ray
- setting
- perhaps surgery and anaesthetic
- plaster or fixing
- pain control
- overnight hotel services
- lavatories and bathing facilities
- meals
- discharge
- outpatient clinics
- physiotherapy and appliances
- and goodness knows what else I have overlooked.

The point is that there are umpteen components to fixing someone up. They are all part of the patient experience, each one of them important and integral to the quality experience. Any one of them can let any of the others down.

Exercise

 Consider one episode of care, for example a patient who breaks his leg in an industrial accident at work. Carry out a mapping exercise to establish the number of interfaces between departments the patient might encounter in the whole experience. Calculate the number of people whom the patient might encounter.

Consider the role of CG in improving the experience and ensuring consistency in treatment for all patients who might go through the same experience.

A hesitant and depressed patient visiting a GP in primary care experiences an intrusive receptionist who makes getting an appointment difficult, 'Is it urgent dear?'; waits in a noisy waiting room full of screaming kids and does not hear his name being called over the tannoy system; can't properly articulate his concerns to the doctor and feels rushed; is sceptical about the drugs he has been prescribed; lives alone; doesn't eat properly; eventually disappears into the hustle and bustle of modern living and becomes forgotten. Who knows what happens to him?

I know, no such thing would ever occur in your practice, but …

Who would deny there is potential for it to happen in any practice that does not realise that the whole patient experience is part of the patient's passage back to optimal function – getting better.

CG is about looking at the whole experience and adding the important dimensions of professional development and sharing best practice. Underpinning all of that is the NHS's new variation on TLC: it is TPC!

Teamwork : Partnership : Communication

Teamwork

In my experience the NHS has had a schizophrenic relationship with team working. Some teams work fabulously well together. Paramedics depend on each other and work for each other. Surgical teams, often working at the most complicated and leading edge of medicine, could only do what they do working as a team.

What's it like where you work? Do you feel part of a team? Delivering CG can only be done when all of the professionals involved in providing care work together as a team. This may mean a whole new approach, particularly in primary care.

At service level, clinical teams analysing and assessing the quality of their services and seeking ways to improve them will be a multi-disciplinary effort. And it is increasingly likely to be a multi-agency activity.

Exercise

 Many patients will have needs, particularly those suffering chronic conditions that require care from a range of health professionals.

Choose an example which crosses the boundaries of primary and secondary care, needing an integrated approach. Examples might be diabetes mellitus, epilepsy or asthma. Consider the role of multi-sectoral, multi-professional care.

It is probably safe to assume that the patient doesn't care too much about where the care comes from, as long as they get it – and seamlessly.

What would you include in a strategy to deliver seamless care, with account-ability linking back to the sponsoring organisations?

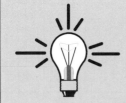

THINK BOX

Against the background of the previous exercise and your conclusions, does the question become one of realistic delivery expectations? Can all these services really work together? Social services have different funding from health, they have different managerial frameworks and are cursed (or blessed) by the intervention of elected members – councillors. In Northern Ireland they are busy demolishing the walls between health and social services and the proposed Northern Ireland Assembly will have control over the services as a joint agency. Is that the solution for the rest of the UK?

Let's talk about the 'untalkable'

Mention the name 'Bristol' in the NHS and professionals freeze and critics reach for their word processors. I feel genuinely sorry for the army of professionals and others working at Bristol. That hospital must now, after all it's been through, be the safest hospital in the world.

Of course it went through tragic times and no one can begin to address how some parents must feel.

However, there is something to be said that is almost unmentionable. Some clinicians working in smaller clinical specialties or at the forefront of medical advances may have few local counterparts with whom they can make comparisons and assess their outcomes and quality.

Let's be clear, I am not entering into a 'right or wrong' debate and I fully understand the issues around whistle blowing and how the medical profession, in times of trouble, tends to close ranks. But the unanswered question is 'would a different approach based on the concepts of CG have made a difference?' Do you want to try and answer that question?

Exercise

 Consider how smaller clinical specialties and sub-specialties could share CG arrangements, either regionally or nationally, to benchmark their performance and improve the quality of what they do.

Pick a specialty (say renal services) and design a system for CG based on improved communication and cascading best practice.

SECTION 4

An invitation you can't refuse!

All NHS organisations are involved in CG and each and every one of them must demonstrate that they are implementing CG procedures – both now and in the future. The Gods of Whitehall do not see this as a one-off thing. CG has a 10-year roll out and is seen as a continuing programme of education and improvement.

The development of CG is focused at local level but there is a national framework of key tasks that all NHS outfits will need to demonstrate progress against. Here they come...

 You may not need to read the whole of the next section. You might take the view that if it's not your organisation or department you need not worry your pretty little head about it. Why should you? You've got enough to worry about with the deluge of all the other stuff the Department of Health throws at you! But it might be worth skimming through the roles and responsibilities of all the others. CG is a joined-up thing and having a feel for everyone else's contribution may not be such a bad thing.

You decide. Your call!

Clinical Governance and the Health Authority

Health authorities

One of the key functions of health authorities is leading the process to compile the Health Improvement Programme, or HImP.

What's a HImP? OK, here's a five minute 'teach-in' on HImPs:

 Health Improvement Programmes or HImPs are at the heart of the Government's aim to recognise the causes of ill health and to do something about it. They are a local action plan to improve health and modernise services in the context of 'joined up services'.

HImPs aim to:

- bring together the local NHS with local authorities and others, including the voluntary sector
- set the strategic framework for improving health
- tackle inequalities
- develop faster, more convenient services of a consistently high standard.

In case this is starting to look like another strategic document that sits on the shelf in a manager's office, HImPs must:

- be action focused
- set out high-level objectives
- summarise the commitments of the local players to deliver
- include measurable targets for improvement
- demonstrate how resources are to be used to improve the health and well being of the population and modernise the NHS.

So, no hiding place!

They must also:

- involve everyone with an interest
- engage PCGs in the strategic planning process, ensuring that the HImP is guided by the perspective and knowledge that they are able to bring to bear (See, you've got a nice mention. Very flattering, now you've got to want to be involved, haven't you?)
- take proper account of locally determined needs
- include national priorities
- enable hospital clinicians to contribute their expertise on how best to meet local needs
- offer the opportunity for the local community and its leaders, e.g. local councillors, to influence the strategy.

So, everyone gets their say on what local health priorities should be.

OK 'teach-in' over ... back to work

You can see from all this that there are a lot of folk, and many services, who can have their say in a HImP. That means plenty of opportunities for what management gurus describe as 'service interface failures'. In other words, too many cooks can make a real mess in the kitchen.

So, health authorities must identify the priorities for quality improvement in the locality through the needs assessment phase of the HImP. How do they do that? Good question!

The answer is by drawing on individual health organisations' action plans and any other sources of information they can lay their hot sweaty hands on!

Exercise

 Devise a process to capture information on PCG, PCG Trust and Trust Hospital action plans for service development.

Consider formal and informal methods and include such sources as annual reports and primary care investment plans. Oh, and a bit of gossip here and there. You know no one in the NHS can keep a secret!

Backing winners

The next job for the health authority is to decide on the investments and actions required to be included in the HImP and to ensure improvements in the quality of services. Picking winners and making investments that will bear fruit as better services.

Exercise

Draw up an investment strategy that would identify services worth investing in and consider what outcome assurances might be required.

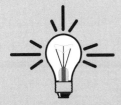

THINK BOX

Are there any lost causes? If a service is not necessarily dangerous but poor, will investing in it necessarily improve it? At what point do you cut your losses? Is withdrawing a service on the grounds of poor quality ever an option for the NHS? The public depends on NHS services. Do services have to be kept going at all costs or any price?

A fountain of knowledge

Health authorities will be working with a diverse group of services across the health and social service spectrum, and with the voluntary sector. As the policy develops, they will accumulate a vast amount of information and knowledge about what's good and where the best practice is.

Their task is to promote good practice based on their experience of working with others.

Exercise

 How would you centralise a health authority's knowledge of good practice? Consider the diverse number of contacts the health authority will have and the difficulties that might present. Then consider how the information could be shared. What methods and processes would you use?

They are new and they're gonna be good!

One of the biggest changes health authorities are managing is the emergence and transition of primary care groups (PCGs). PCGs are new and complex organisations. They will take some time to find their feet. Health authorities have a role in the development of CG in PCGs.

Exercise

PCGs are home for a diverse number of professionals: doctors, nurses, professions allied to medicine, managers and administration staff as well as the voluntary sector.

Consider the variety of professions, training, background and levels of awareness and understanding.

How would a health authority support CG in those circumstances? Consider such options as training, conferencing, newsletters, benchmarking and other management tools available to facilitate CG and continuing professional development in the PCG environment.

Widows and orphans

The health authority has a special position in that it can see across service boundaries. Therefore it is in a position to identify those services that have insufficient critical mass to undertake CG on a purely local basis. They must ensure adequate arrangements are put in place.

Exercise

Make a list of the specialist services that occupy a niche in the overall service framework. How do you identify them? Can you use cost (or revenue) as the factor or is the number of patients seen a better yardstick? Specialist services are rarely the least expensive services. Neither do they see the most people.

Once identified, how would you make adequate arrangements to ensure they were involved in CG initiatives?

Start in your own back yard!

Health authorities remain responsible for some vital services, such as public health, communicable disease control and health needs assessment, as well as providing clinical advice. The health authority is responsible for the CG of these services.

Exercise

 Take one of the health authority functions and consider the factors contributing to its CG. List them and devise an approach to ensure the benchmarking of the service and the continuing professional development of the staff involved.

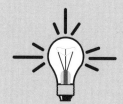

THINK BOX

One of the professions that became rather eclipsed during the health reforms of the 90s is public health.

They must be feeling that their time has come again. After all, CG with its reliance on audit, evidence-based decision making and guidelines is very close to what the 'smarties' in public health have been telling us to do all along.

Should public health people be leading this process? Is there any room for the manager at all? After all, who better to sort out a doc than another doc armed to the teeth with the evidence?

Clinical Governance and the Primary Care Group

Primary care groups

Some say it is easier to get good habits into an organisation that is being set up from scratch, than it is to teach an old dog new tricks … maybe. I guess we'll know in a year or two once PCGs have had a chance to find out which way up they are!

CG is to play a big part in their setting up and development. There are four steps which are key to the implementation:

1 establishing leadership, accountability and working arrangements
2 carrying out a baseline assessment of capacity and capability
3 formulating an action plan in the light of the assessment
4 clarifying reporting arrangements for CG within the Board.

The four steps to heaven, of which more later (steps that is, not heaven!).

PCGs will probably spend a year settling into their new roles and responsibilities. It is important for any new organisation to set itself reasonable targets and to have modest ambitions. In some places expectations will be high, in others failure will be welcomed.

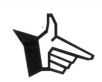

It is important for any new organisation to set itself reasonable targets and to have modest ambitions.

We all know the emergence of PCGs has left some former fundholders disappointed, has put pressures on the workforce and created a great deal of uncertainty for many staff. On the other hand, they have been welcomed by others who have seized the opportunity to create new working partnerships with new colleagues.

Wherever you sit in the argument, there is a job to be done. Underpinning the success of what any PCG might achieve is the concept of CG: a way to bind services together with the triple threads of quality, education and improving practice.

So, with all the other distractions that embryo organisations face, don't forget the fast evolving world of CG.

What's new?

Exercise

Create a system where new CG guidance can be quickly evaluated and implemented into a PCG. Is it a job for a single person or should there be a multi-disciplinary group to review new CG guidance and disseminate it? What's your approach?

Split personality?

PCGs are both providers and commissioners of healthcare. That puts them in a unique position. They have a dual responsibility to ensure the CG of their services and to safeguard the CG of the services delivered by others on their behalf.

Exercise

Try to list the full range of services commissioned by a PCG – headline specialties will do for now. What steps can you take to ensure the CG of those services? How would you arrange to play a part in the CG development of those services in the future?

We're in this together

PCGs are intended to be a multi-sector, multi-agency forum providing seamless services across department and functional boundaries. Health will be jointly responsible for social and other services **and** social services will be jointly responsible for the CG of health.

This creates a whole new meaning to the phrase 'working together'.

Exercise

 List the issues that arise from multi-agency, joint accountability for CG. Take into account the variation in management arrangements between agencies and their levels of quality at the moment. How would you address them?

Let's be frank ...

Multi-agency working will take some getting used to. Many primary care teams will already have a good record of working alongside social services but this is different. Working alongside is one thing, working with, sharing budgets and being jointly responsible is quite another. CG puts pressure on all health providers to increase the levels of quality and service. Improving quality depends on a frank admission of what the level of service is like now. It is difficult enough to get colleagues whom you may have worked with for years to admit they might be able to perform better. Getting strangers to do it is a whole new ball game.

The situation is further complicated by the fact that the Commission for Health Improvement (CHImP) is going to be judgemental about your CG programme. Mmmm ... yes, judgemental, a word right out of DoH guidance. Mmmm indeed!

Exercise

 What steps can you take to establish an open relationship with new colleagues, to encourage them to be frank about their services?

How will your organisation react to the arrival of CHImP? How could you prepare your organisation not to feel threatened by the arrival of CHImP, and to see it as a learning exercise?

CG is not just for Christmas, it's for life!

CG is a process of continuous development. That means:

'Things can only get better'

... now where have I heard that before?

Anyway, I can hear you say 'Yeah, yeah, we know it is continuing and all that. So what?' Well there is an important issue here. PCGs commission services, don't they? And some of those services will be on the basis of long-term service agreements. Get the picture?

If you are not very careful, services commissioned on long-term agreements could turn into a CG relic. Over time, clinical practice may change and approaches to treatments may vary or improve. If a service is commissioned over, say, a five-year period, what about taking into account the improvements that might emerge during the five-year currency of the service agreement?

Exercise

What principles would you apply to long-term service agreements to ensure that CG – particularly continuous improvement – is delivered throughout the agreement period?

Exercise

 Not all of the services commissioned by a PCG will come from the NHS. Some may come from the private sector. Are there any differences to be considered when applying the principles of CG to the private sector? What are they?

No visible means of support

What about Primary Care Act Pilots? Remember them! PCGs may have member practitioners working in the pilots. Applying the principles of CG in the pilots and supporting the professionals working there is just as important as elsewhere in the NHS.

Exercise

What are the special considerations in applying CG to the delivery of general medical services and personal medical services in Primary Care Act Pilots?

Clinical Governance and the NHS Trust

NHS Trusts

NHS Trusts have the same responsibility as PCGs for undertaking the four main implementation steps.

To save you the bother of flipping back through half a dozen pages to find out what they are, here with no expense spared they are printed again:

1 establishing leadership, accountability and working arrangements
2 carrying out a baseline assessment of capacity and capability
3 formulating an action plan in the light of the assessment
4 clarifying reporting arrangements for CG within the Board.

The four steps to heaven, of which more later (steps that is, not heaven!).

By now, you should be able to recite 'the four steps to heaven' off by heart. It's not difficult. Think of it this way:

1 find someone who's prepared to put their head on the block to achieve it
2 find out how bad things really are (or good)
3 figure out what you can do about it
4 and let the boss know, so he can make sure you do it.

Easy, everyday management in the NHS … ho, ho!

What else?

Get everyone marching in step

Many secondary services will have services provided by tertiary referral or others outside the Trust.

CG applies across the board and the commissioner is as responsible for the CG of the services as is the services supplier him/herself.

Exercise

Devise a system to ensure the CG of services commissioned from tertiary and other services.

Keep up, keep up

Trusts are complex places. They have an enormous range of services and a huge variety of professionals and disciplines working in them. CG applies across the board. Developing a programme of CG to comply with existing guidance may be difficult enough. Keeping up-to-date with developments is a gargantuan job.

Exercise

 Devise a system that allows for the development of a CG programme and takes into account the possibility of future guidance, allowing flexibility for changes.

Consider an approach on a segmented, departmental basis, a specialty basis or a Trust-wide initiative.

What are the pluses and minuses of each approach and what would your preferred option be?

Look out for 'tribalising' a system and the dangers of 'disaggregating' the effort. CG is supposed to bring people together. Remember all that 'joined up ness'?

Everyone has to play this game

In the past, some medics have been a touch reluctant (ha!) to take part in national clinical audits or Confidential Inquiries. If we are to learn from each other we need to know what is going on. So the days of medics hiding their good deeds are over. Everybody has to play the game.

Exercise

 Consider why some medics have declined to participate in national clinical audits or Confidential Inquiries.

– Is it a time thing?
– Is it because they don't think they are really 'confidential'?
– Do they see no benefit in doing it?

What do you consider to be the reasons?

How would you encourage medical colleagues to play their part and contribute to this vital national resource of knowledge, experience and learning?

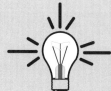 **THINK BOX**

Is this just another stick to beat doctors with? We are quick to blame the medical profession when things go wrong. Doctors do live in a threatened environment, don't they? Or should we be more ruthless with the medical professional and consider a failure to participate in national clinical audits or Confidential Inquiries as serious professional misconduct?

If you're in a mess, we are in a mess too!

NHS Trusts have to do more than ensure CG in the services they commission on behalf of others. Guidance makes them jointly responsible for the CG of services that are delivered on a multi-sector, multi-agency basis. Oh, yes they are!

Exercise

Consider one multi-agency service a Trust might be involved in. Take examples such as discharge or dementia services.

Consider what are the joint responsibilities for CG in delivering the seamless service to the patient. Devise a method of outcome accountability for all of the services involved.

Off-sick has arrived ...

For the want of a better expression the NHS has a new regulatory body. The water companies have Off-wat, the phone companies have Off-tel and the NHS has the Commission for Health Improvement.

Otherwise known as:

Off-sick!

Well, not really, but you know what I mean.

This is the first time the NHS has had a regulatory body with the power to descend on an NHS establishment and examine its performance. Some people have welcomed it as a development that can only help to leverage up performance and quality. Others see it as the arrival of the 'health police'. Mmm, this is not going to be easy to manage. CHImP *will* make judgements about the performance of the Trust.

Exercise

 Develop a Trust-wide strategy to prepare the organisation for the arrival of CHImP.

How would you create a welcoming and open attitude, based on forming learning relationships with people who could very well be critical about the quality of services of the CG programme?

Clinical Governance and the Regional Offices of the NHS Executive

Regional Offices of the NHS Executive

See, I told you everybody is doing it! Even the Regional Offices have a part to play in the implementation and development of CG.

They have three main tasks:

1 ensuring all guidance is implemented in a coherent manner
2 assessing year-on-year progress against an individual organisation's objectives for the four key steps – you must know what they are by now but in case you can't call them to mind, or haven't got the strength left to turn back the pages and find out, here they are again:

   - establishing leadership, accountability and working arrangements
   - carrying out a baseline assessment of capacity and capability
   - formulating an action plan in the light of the assessment
   - clarifying reporting arrangements for CG within the Board.

   The four steps to heaven, of which more later. (Steps that is, not heaven!)

3 facilitating links between the Commission for Health Improvement (Off-sick) and NHS organisations, and making sure NHS organisations develop and implement action plans following CHImP reviews or investigations.

THINK BOX

There may only be three tasks but they are very big ones! They all come into the performance management category. There will be a vast number of NHS organisations in every Region that will be a mix of types. Won't performance managing these three headings take an army of people? Is this what the Government has in mind? If Regions are put under managerial unit cost pressures – which is highly likely – how will the Regions deliver? Will this be management in name only? Can we expect to see this whole process gather dust someplace? Will the Government be prepared to fund the whole CG process? New money or from savings?

Exercise

 Devise a cost-effective method of ensuring the implementation of guidance across a Region. Consider reporting systems, the use of technology and personal visits. What are the cost and man-power implications?

Picking up the pieces

Think for a moment about an organisation that has had a visit from CHImP and has been found 'wanting'. Oh dear! There are implications for morale, professional pride and managerial integrity. This could turn ugly. Regions are responsible for picking up the pieces. That is to say, making sure the recommendations of CHImP are implemented.

Exercise

 What factors would you take into account in implementing the recommendations of CHImP following an unfavourable review or investigation? Consider how you would approach the issues of organisational morale, the potential for the migration of good staff leaving to work in other organisations, and professional pride. How would you go about getting back the organisation's self-belief?

Is it a CHImP or a Gorilla?

A great deal of CG's success depends on the success of CHImP. No one yet knows how the first visits from CHImP will be received. Some say they will be welcomed, others are already calling the CHImP a Gorilla. That is to say:

GO and **R**oot out **ILL**egal **A**cts

How CHImP does what it does is as important as what it does. Let's have a closer look at exactly what it is they are supposed to be doing.

The first responsibility is to the taxpayer and the boss, the Secretary of State. Here's what the NHS Guidance on the topic has to say:

> 'CHImP will have the key role in providing the public and the Secretary of State with the assurance that CG is being implemented appropriately at every level of the NHS.'

Sounds easy doesn't it! What do they do for an encore? Well, there are five other core functions.

Let's have a look.

1 Provide national leadership and develop and disseminate CG principles

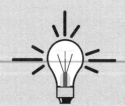

THINK BOX

The issue of leadership is worth focusing on. The dictionary defines 'leadership' as influence but it also provides another synonym: 'authority'.

It is easy to mix up the two. Some will see CHImP as influencing change, others will see it as using its authority to make change happen. How do you see it? Is the difference important? Why?

Anyway, back to the reality.

2 **Independently scrutinise local CG arrangements to support, promote and deliver high-quality services, through a rolling programme of local reviews of service providers**

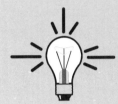

THINK BOX

A rolling programme. What does that mean to you? Apparently, every Trust can expect a visit every 3–4 years. Doesn't that seem like a long time? Most independent quality assurance outfits will visit an accredited unit once a year.

A lot can happen in 48 months – a lot that is good and a lot that is bad too. Should the visits be more frequent? What are the resource implications?

Schools have a visit from Off-sted every so often and they are already moaning about the amount of time it takes to prepare for a visit and the stress it causes. Is the NHS in for a similar experience? Will it all be worth it? How will we know?

3 **Undertake a programme of service reviews to monitor national implementation of National Service Frameworks and review progress locally on implementation of these Frameworks and NICE Guidance**

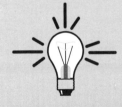

THINK BOX

Given the range of expertise involved in the spread of services offered by the NHS and the fact that CG is common to them all, where will CHImP get the expertise from to make the service reviews meaningful? Will CHImP be full of 'know nothings' or 'has beens'? Who will consider it a career move to work at CHImP?

Also bear in mind that this is likely to be professionals reviewing professionals – does this move on up at all?

4 Help the NHS identify and tackle serious or persistent clinical problems

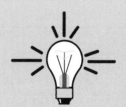

THINK BOX

The Commission will have the capacity for rapid investigation and intervention to help put problems right but aren't there as many issues about resources as anything else? If all these experts are going to fly around the place putting everything right, wouldn't they be better off seeing patients or running something properly in the first place? Will they be full time with CHImP, sitting in the crew room ready to helicopter into some luckless Trust that has fouled-up? Or will they be working folk who will have to leave their day job for a week or two to go and sort someone else's mess out? What happens to their workload in the meantime?

5 Take on responsibility for overseeing and assisting with external incident enquiries

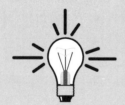

THINK BOX

This is the real tough job. This is the job that is done when all else fails or something serious has gone wrong.

If CHImP is to provide leadership and coax the NHS down the path of CG, is this a job too far?

Should it be done by another agency? Or at the very least fire-walled from CHImP's regular work?

So now you know what CHImP will do. There's a lot to think about, isn't there? We can only wish colleagues who end up working there, the very best of British luck!

SECTION 5

OK, what about the real stuff? What have we got to do?

The four key steps revealed

Yes folks, it's time to 'do' the four steps to heaven. Let's see if you've been paying attention. Write below, what they are:

1

2

3

4

Can't do it, eh. Well for the last time I'll tell you, turn over the page …

The four steps to heaven

1 Establishing leadership, accountability and working arrangements.
2 Carrying out a baseline assessment of capacity and capability.
3 Formulating an action plan in the light of the assessment.
4 Clarifying reporting arrangements for CG within the Board.

Now, that's the last time I'm going to help you remember this. For goodness sake, cut round the edges and stick it on the wall! They are a very important part of CG and the four steps that every health service organisation has to go through as part of embedding CG into their operations.

All the previous stuff has been the vision thing – these are the practical steps you must take in the first year.

Let's take them one at a time and consider what they mean and how we go about doing the 'embedding' bit …

Establishing leadership, accountability and working arrangements

The new NHS Act places a duty of quality on every PCG and NHS Trust. The buck stops with the Chief Executive and the Board.

In practical terms, the Chief Executive will identify a lead clinician who will be responsible for CG in the organisation. Who the lead clinician is will vary from organisation to organisation.

However, make no mistake, it is a pivotal role.

So, the first question is, how does the lead clinician get selected, chosen or press-ganged?

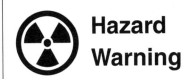

Hazard Warning

As this is so important, shouldn't the head of CG be a member of the Board?

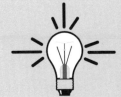

THINK BOX

How should the person be selected and will it make a difference? People's motives make a difference to how they do a job.

1 As the Chief Executive carries the can, should they just pick the person they trust?

2 Should the Board decide?

3 A volunteer may be genuinely keen on the issue and come to the job with enthusiasm that may turn them into a zealot.

4 A press-ganged person may do as little as possible.

5 Was there a ballot?

6 Was the post advertised, internally?

7 Does anyone know how the person was selected?

8 Does it matter?

Is the post holder there to give the Chief Executive some peace of mind or to provide leadership to the organisation? Can you have both?

Exercise

 Consider the role of medical director and the lead person on clinical governance.

• What are the potentials for conflict?

• Should the two posts be held by one person or two?

• What are the benefits and problems in amalgamating the role?

• Aren't many medical director posts part-time? Can they do three jobs?

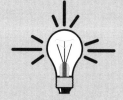 **THINK BOX**

What are they doing in other places? In Northern and Yorkshire Region the lead on CG looks like this:

• 16 Trusts have named the Medical Director
• 11 Trusts have named the Nurse Director
• 2 Trusts have named the Chief Executive
• 5 Trusts have identified a partnership between nurse and medical director.

Are they right? How would you do it?

Being responsible for CG in a large Trust is as complex a job as being the head of CG in a PCG is a sensitive one. It's not rocket science and we can see that the head of CG won't be able to do the whole job on his/her own and he/she will need support. Consider the number of specialties and professions involved. No one could know everything about everything.

Exercise

✔ Design a team to support the head of CG in a NHS Trust and a PCG. Highlight the differences in the models and explain why.

NHS Trust

Board

| Chief Executive

| Medical Director

PCG

Board

| Chairman

Differences:

Whatever the management model, leadership is the key element. You may not be the head of CG (you lucky person), you may be part of the team, or just an interested bystander. Whatever you are, you will have a stake in the success of the role and the implementation of CG.

Let's take time to look at the key elements of successful leadership in the CG process.

Inclusivity

Keeping everyone feeling part of the game.

Exercise

How will you ensure that all the key groups in the organisation are involved and kept fully informed on the purpose and progress of CG? Can you devise a system that doesn't involve everyone forgetting what a patient looks like because they are spending all their time at briefings? And can you come up with a system that doesn't drown everyone in paper?

Commitment from the top

The issue of seniority of the head of CG comes into consideration. If the head of CG is not a member of the Board, free access to the Board is vital.

Having access to the Chief Executive and the Board is something that most people you work with would like to have!

Some organisations are more open than others. Some of the work of CG will be routine and some of the work may involve uncovering poor practice and mistakes. If the medical director is a practising clinician and he or she falls foul of the CG programme, you could have a real mess on your hands.

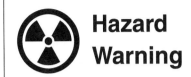

Hazard Warning

Some of the work of CG will be routine and some of the work may involve uncovering poor practice and mistakes. If the medical director is a practising clinician and he or she falls foul of the CG programme, you could have a real mess on your hands.

Exercise

Devise a protocol that would allow the head of CG barrier-free access to the Board and the Chief Executive. Consider the extent to which existing reporting mechanisms and protocols need to be preserved, and the effect that direct access for one person/department might have on other members of staff who consider they have just as important issues they would like to bring to the attention of the Board.

Good external relationships

We already know that CG doesn't begin and end at the boundaries of the organisations we work in. CG overlaps all the contacts we have with the suppliers of other services and organisations we work with. Whoever leads on CG will become the face of CG for your organisation.

They may even become the face of your organisation. For certain, they will become a powerful and influential figure outside the organisation. Indeed, if they do the job well, they could become better known than the medical director and the chief executive. That may not be what the boss had in mind!

Leaving aside the personal issues (much too difficult!) there is a huge task for the head of CG to get to grips with the multitude of outside organisations and interfaces they will be responsible for forging links with.

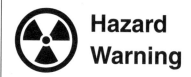

Hazard Warning

For certain, they will become a powerful and influential figure outside the organisation. Indeed, if they do the job well, they could become better known than the medical director and the chief executive. That may not be what the boss had in mind!

Exercise

Devise an induction programme for the head of CG where you work. Who do you consider to be the key players and stakeholders they should meet and what would be the objectives?

Constancy of purpose

Nice phrase, isn't it? It isn't mine. I borrowed it from Department of Health guidance, *Constancy of Purpose.* Lovely phrase, isn't it? Biblical even. What does it mean? Well, I think it means staying focused and keeping this monster we now call CG going in the right direction. CG in complex organisations can easily get lost.

When it comes to purpose, it is about motivation, clarity of vision and single mindedness.

Now you can begin to see why the selection of the right person to lead CG is so important. You don't need a woolly thinker and you can equally do without a zealot. This is a really tough medical challenge – is it fair on a doctor who has no management background to expect him/her to deliver this?

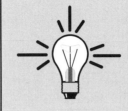

THINK BOX

Now you can begin to see why the selection of the right person to lead CG is so important.

You don't need a woolly thinker and you can equally do without a zealot.

This is a really tough medical challenge – is it fair on a doctor who has no management background to expect him/her to deliver this?

Exercise

Develop an outcomes audit to ensure that CG stays on track. What do you consider to be the key deliverables this year, next year and the year after?

Accounting for progress

In other words, where are we? This is different to measuring outcomes and it is important not to confuse the two. Let me explain.

The lucky person who buys a Ferrari, drives it up the M1 to Birmingham with the CD playing some favourite tracks, the cruise control keeping the speed to exactly 70 mph and the air conditioning adjusting the temperature in the car to a comfortable 65°, is having a great outcome. But if they are supposed to be going to Brighton, they're not making very good progress!

You can have good outcomes but still not make very good progress.

Exercise

✔ Describe a system that would allow the organisation to see, at all times, a comprehensive overview of the progress of the CG programme.

Communication

How many times do we hear that word in the NHS? I'm fed up with it. Communication is generally the answer to most problems and the thing we are all least good at.

CG will hold some real fears for some staff. I've never met anyone who works in the NHS who didn't want to do their best. The trouble is, people often don't know if their best is the right best and if their best can be bettered. CG is much more likely to be a worry to a conscientious member of staff than the laggard. So an important part of CG is to turn it into a stepping stone and not a mill stone.

Any new policy needs policy champions, folk who can see the benefits and will 'champion' the idea into the organisation. Good communication is at the heart of finding and encouraging the 'champions'.

Communication is vital. I hate to use such a cliché but it really is vital. Any new policy needs policy champions, folk who can see the benefits and will 'champion' the idea in the organisation. Good communication is at the heart of finding and encouraging the 'champions'.

Exercise

All staff in the organisation need to know what the CG gurus are up to and what progress is being made. The CG gurus will want to publish some 'quick-wins' to show that their programme is delivering. People outside the organisation will stand ready to be informed about all the good stuff that is going on.

Consider the communication need of the CG group and devise a communications strategy to keep everyone, inside and outside the organisation, in touch with what is going on.

THINK BOX

If the CG group uncovers something nasty, what are the communication issues? Who gets told what and when?

Accountability

All NHS organisations are included in the CG initiative and all of them are obliged to establish clear accountability and working arrangements for CG. Many NHS Trusts have already established a quality committee, they now need to realise that that is not quite the same as CG and they may need to consider whether or not changes in its terms of reference are required.

Exercise

 Consider the composition of a CG committee. Without turning the committee into a group of people of the size that Moses led out of the desert, how would you ensure the committee represents an appropriate balance of skills and interests **and** how best to include public and user input?

Connecting the public into high level discussions about public services may seem like a novel idea in the NHS, but industry has been talking to its customers for years. Perhaps we should try it!

Now let's move on to the second step.

Carrying out a baseline assessment of capacity and capability

Just how good are you over at your place? I guess we need to find out. Think of it as a kind of stock take. The so-called baseline assessment is a foundation job for the first year of CG. This job needs to be done well as it will form part of the development planning for subsequent years.

PCGs may well find this exercise a bit onerous and may be short of the special skills it needs. Ask the health authority for some help.

The process should be organisation wide and participative. Mmm, easier said than done.

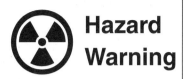 **Hazard Warning**

This is no time to pretend, cover up or be shy. This is a time for some stripped pine honesty. Make out that a service is better than it is and you run the risk of missing out on development cash to sort it out, and the embarrassment of the service tipping over when it is under pressure.

Exercise

 A searching and honest analysis of your organisation's strengths and weaknesses in relation to current performance on quality is at the heart of what is required. Expect there to be some sensitivities around admitting what's not so good and expect some boasting about what is average! The good stuff will be obvious.

How would you go about this part of the job and create an atmosphere that encourages frankness and openness? What part might anonymity play? Public confessions might be good for the soul but will they get the job done?

How will you know if something is good, or not?

Perceptions of quality vary. Something might be technically good, excellent even, but if it is delivered in shoddy surroundings by morose staff, the patient perception may be that it is not a quality service. Similarly, a relatively poor service can be popular with patients because of the manner of its delivery. Staff are pleasant, jolly and the clinic runs to time. So, what's quality?

Exercise

✔ Develop a way of identifying problematic services that is a balance of objective data and feedback from service users.

Can you trust the data?

I guess a better question is, are there any data? Monitoring performance is fundamental to CG and the roles of data capture, data store and data access are pretty obvious.

Exercise

How would you assess the current data available to you in terms of its validity and accuracy? What reference points would you develop to test the data?

Are there some invisible faultlines?

CG looks across the whole of the organisation's effectiveness. Deficits in key mechanisms may not be apparent at the moment but as CG places greater pressures on the organisation, they may become apparent at some awkward moments. Best to check this out, don't you think?

Exercise

 Consider the hidden, key mechanisms of your organisation, such as for risk management and multi-disciplinary clinical audit, information management and patient input in policy and care protocols.

Take one of the mechanisms and develop the principles required to audit its performance in order to establish any shortcomings.

'Joined-up-ness'

I very much hope my newly invented word finds a permanent place in the lexicon of healthcare because it sums up what otherwise might take several paragraphs to explain. Something as potentially all embracing and complex as CG might turn out to need more than its fair share of 'joined-up-ness'.

Exercise

What steps need to be taken, as foundation actions, to ensure the integration of the organisation's activities with its systems?

Whilst we are on the subject of 'joined-up-ness', there is the little matter of the HImP. (In case you've forgotten what that is, there is a quick overview on page 32 to this [see also Section 4].)

Exercise

Think about establishing explicit links with HImPs and NSFs and other local priorities. The question is really about where the horse fits into the cart. I guess a horse could push a cart but it is better if it pulls one. So where is the push-pull relationship here? Consider which process is driving CG – initiatives or priorities? Does it matter? What are the consequences of the wrong process driving the process? (If you see what I mean!)

It's not me, it's the others...

Think about these four headings:

1 information management and technology (IM&T)
2 human resources (HR)
3 continuing professional development (CPD)
4 research and development (R&D).

They are all groups that spend a great deal of money and some are departments in their own right. They all make a major contribution to an organisation's success and they all have a role to play in CG: IM&T for data and other obvious contributions; HR representing staff, the largest resource and the biggest revenue cost centre and the ones who deliver the good and the bad services; CPD at the heart of the continuum that is CG; and R&D that leads us to improvements and new approaches.

Exercise

 Consider the four headings and design ways in which underpinning strategies will connect them to the CG process and support CG initiatives within the organisation.

Is it deliverable? Otherwise known as the reality check

It's easy to get excited about quality isn't it? Service is seductive. As far as I can see, CG doesn't arrive in a big box with a pretty pink ribbon and a bundle of money.

Quite the opposite.

CG, it seems to me, must be delivered largely within the existing cost envelope. Put that harrowing news against our understanding of human behaviour and, more particularly NHS folk's behaviour, and you may have some trouble brewing.

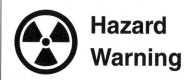

Hazard Warning

Everyone in the organisation will get the idea that something good is going to happen to them, and in their department. And it ain't, well not immediately and maybe not for some time.

Ask the questions: do you want to do the job better, be better at what you do and improve? The overwhelming answer will be, not half!

The NHS staff are a curious lot. Survey after survey enquiring into staff wish lists, put continuing professional development alongside (if not higher) than more money.

So, if you are going to rush around the organisation talking-up quality and enthusing everyone with ideas about doing things better, you're going to have to deal with what the management gurus call 'increased expectations'.

Everyone in the organisation will get the idea that something good is going to happen to them, and in their department. And you and I know it ain't, well not immediately and maybe not for some time.

Decisions will have to be made about what is feasible and what isn't. What is achievable and what isn't. There is nothing more likely to derail CG than a lot of ambitious plans that are left to go rusty.

Exercise

 When a quality initiative has a significant resource significance, how do you decide priorities?

Consider a method of determining priorities that is fair and transparent and likely to be acceptable, even to the disappointed.

Take into account the role of the HImP and other agreed priorities and the part they might play in determining what is feasible and what is not.

Let's cheer everyone up

Let's not depress ourselves with the thought that everything in the baseline assessment is bad, or that the whole thing is a pile of worms. There will be good things and there will be some bad things.

Exercise

Consider ways of briefing everyone in the organisation with the outcome of the baseline survey.

Look at making it a motivational experience highlighting what is good but at the same time taking what is less good as an opportunity to improve. Consider using milestones for improvement.

Ready for step three.

Formulating and agreeing a development plan

OK, so now we know how good (or bad) the organisation is, what do we do next? Well, the answer is another plan! On the basis of the baseline assessment, the idea is to put together a plan for developing CG and addressing such sexy topics as:

Closing the gap

Or put another way, closing the gap between the present performance of a service, or part of the organisation, to where you think it should be.

Exercise

 Consider a service where the baseline assessment reveals less than optimal performance. What bearing does the level of performance have on the remedial and training measures you may need to take?

Think about the steps you might take to improve performance. Will a visit to a better performing unit do the trick? Is professional education indicated? Is there an obvious under resourcing at the heart of the problem?

At what point do you say, 'we are not good enough at this and we won't do it at all'?

Time for some cross-addressing

We know, or we should by now, that CG is everybody's business and we have thought about the role played by IM&T colleagues, the HR department, organisational structures, CPD and cross-linkages with other organisations. So let's get joining-up …

Exercise

Describe the organisational infrastructure required to allow for the cross-flow of information and ideas, to link up the various parts of the organisation in the CG programme.

Does everyone really, really understand all this?

Most likely the baseline assessment will have shown up the need for some staff training. Don't forget, staff are the folk who deliver the services at the sharp end and they'd better know and be signed up to what is going on, or you might just as well go and do a more useful job, such as cleaning the catseyes on the M1.

Exercise

  Pick one of the following headings:

1 staff education and training
2 personal development plans
3 Board member induction
4 clinical training skills for clinicians
5 management skills for clinicians

and identify how you would respond to development needs.

Don't get carried away

The backbone planning document is the HImP. Everything in your development plans should link closely to both the HImP and, as they emerge, National Service Frameworks.

Exercise

It is easy to pay lip service to linkages with HImPs and NSFs. Don't, they are important documents.

How would you tie development plans into them and what measure could you use to test the outcomes?

Nearly there – this is the last step.

Clarifying reporting arrangements

Telling the Board how great you are (or not) and, by the way, everyone else.

What you tell the Board, what the Board wants to know and the nature and range of the CG issues that are taken to the Board, will be crucial to the development of the process as a whole.

All NHS Boards now have their meetings in public and the agenda for the meeting is published. So who sees the agenda?

- The whole organisation.
- The local media.
- The public.
- The organisation's partners.

The content of the agenda will send a powerful signal to them all. The more searching and substantial the issues discussed by the Board, the more it will be concluded that the organisation knows what it is doing and is taking CG seriously.

Exercise

Consider the content of a CG report to the Board that castigates a service or contains information that could undermine public confidence in a service.

There are mechanisms for Boards to legitimately take such an item privately (HSG 207/1998 provides guidance). However, what steps could you take to present the information to the media without disrupting public confidence and causing an outcry? Consider off-the-record briefings with journalists or engaging the services of a professional PR company. Could you look for help from politicians and patient groups?

The Annual Report

From 2000 onwards Trusts, HAs, PCGs and PCTs will have a new job to do. They must publish an annual CG report. What goes into it?

The Department of Health has been kind enough to say that the style and detailed content of annual reports is a 'matter for local determination'. I think they mean it's up to you.

However, they are not best pleased with glossy brochures that cost the earth and use money that should be spent doing hip operations or something useful. If you are proud of your achievements and want to look like a professional outfit, why not do the best job you can without going over the top.

Here are some ground rules:

1 keep the language simple, no doctor jargon or management speak
2 think about translations for minority languages, taped versions for the blind and special needs patients
3 use quantitative data as a way of showing progress and present it in an easily understandable form – lots of pie charts and stuff like that
4 compare your performance by using the NHS Performance Assessment Frameworks and the High Level Performance Indicators.

Try and approach the publication from the basics and cover the following points in a straightforward way:

1 where did we start from? (the baseline calculation)
2 what progress have we made and how do we know?
3 what happens next? (the action plan for next year).

In later years, you may have had a visit from Off-sick (CHImP) and their report should be included in your report.

What else? Well the detail should cover:

Who's going to write this segment?

- An explanation of the leadership, accountability and working arrangements for implementing clinical governance.
- Work to ensure that clinical decision making is increasingly evidence based. This should include local action as well as progress on implementation of National Service Framework and NICE guidelines.
- Progress on integrated planning for quality including information establishing explicit links to HImPs and, where appropriate, National Service Frameworks.
- Progress on Continuing Professional Development and lifelong learning, and on designing ways in which staff development, educational and workforce solutions are being used to support clinical governance.
- Participation in, and impact of, multi-disciplinary clinical audit programmes, including national specialty and sub-specialty audits (and National Confidential Enquiries).
- The identification of particular services in which there are identified shortfalls in quality and of deficits in other clinical governance support mechanisms (e.g. risk management, clinical audit).
- Evidence of active working with the public, users of services and their carers.
- An account of the mechanisms that have been established to ensure that lessons are being learned from complaints, adverse incidents and enquiries into services.

So what are you waiting for? That's the four steps – welcome to heaven!

There is just one more thing

Monitoring

You didn't think they'd let you get away without monitoring, did you! What would all the people at Region do?

Region has the primary responsibility for monitoring CG arrangements, performance management and its implementation in NHS Trusts and HAs. It will be looking for year-on-year improvements.

HAs will be in the firing line as the first line monitor for CG in PCGs and Trusts.

The new NHS Performance Assessment Framework will complement the introduction of CG by focusing on the quality and effectiveness of healthcare, as well as on efficiency.

Oh, yes. Then there is the Commission for Health Improvement. Well, we know all about them. They're Off-sick – enough said.

The final monitor will be the self-regulatory arrangements for health professionals that are supposed to be 'closely' aligned to CG.

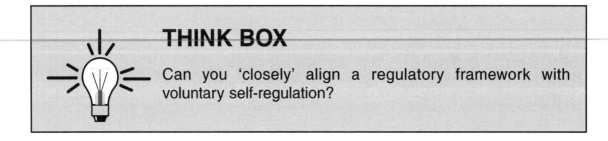

THINK BOX

Can you 'closely' align a regulatory framework with voluntary self-regulation?

Four steps to heaven
Action Plan

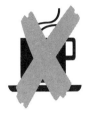

No!

Sorry, no time for coffee. Here's what you've got to do and by when.

Who will do it?

How?

April 1999

Health authorities, Trusts, PCGs and PCTs should have identified lead clinicians for CG and set up appropriate structures, reflecting DoH guidance.

NHS Trusts should have set up Board sub-committees for overseeing CG in their own organisations.

By September 1999

Baseline assessments carried out in accordance with guidance. Trusts and HAs should agree with their Regional Office a process and timescale for conducting the assessments. PCGs and PCTs to agree similar arrangements with their HA.

Following on

In line with guidance, produce and begin to implement agreed development plan for CG locally. The plan should include the activities and timescales for 'closing the gap', developing infrastructure, staff and Board development, planning and prioritisation and, where appropriate, milestones to assist in assessing achievement.

Who will do it?

How?

Trust and HA monitoring should form part of the existing performance management process.

PCGs and PCTs: a process should be agreed with the HA.

On going

Organisations should ensure they have appropriate mechanisms in place to deliver routine Board reports on progress made in implementing CG. The reports should reflect guidance and look to both the short and medium term.

Annually

HAs, PCGs, PCTs and Trusts should produce reports on what they are doing to improve and maintain clinical quality.

Clinical governance at a glance

Who does it affect?	Trust	HA	PCG	PCT
1 Clear lines of responsibility and accountability for the overall quality of clinical care:				
• The NHS Trust Chief Executive carries the ultimate responsibility for assuring the quality of services provided by the Trust.	✓			✓
• A designated senior clinician is responsible for ensuring that systems for clinical governance are in place and for monitoring their continued effectiveness.	✓	✓	✓	✓
• Formal arrangements for NHS Trust, PCT and PCG Boards to discharge their responsibilities for clinical quality through a clinical governance committee.	✓		✓	✓
• Regular reports to NHS Boards on the quality of clinical care given the same importance as monthly financial reports.	✓		✓	✓
• An annual report on clinical governance.	✓	✓	✓	✓

Who does it affect?	Trust	HA	PCG	PCT
2 A comprehensive programme of quality improvement activities which includes:				
• Full participation by all hospital doctors in audit programmes including specialty and sub-specialty national audit programmes endorsed by the Commission for Health Improvement.	✓	✓		
• Full participation in the current four National Confidential Enquiries.	✓	✓		
• Evidence-based practice is supported and applied routinely in everyday practice.	✓	✓	✓	✓
• Ensuring the clinical standards of National Service Frameworks and NICE recommendations are implemented.	✓	✓	✓	✓
• Workforce planning and development (i.e. recruitment and retention of appropriately trained workforce) is fully integrated within the NHS organisation's service planning.	✓	✓	✓	✓
• Continuing Professional Development programmes aimed at meeting the development needs of individual health professionals and the service needs of the organisation are in place and supported locally.	✓	✓	✓	✓
• Appropriate safeguards to govern access to, and storage of, confidential patient information as recommended in the Caldicott Report on the Review of Patient-identifiable Information.	✓	✓	✓	✓

Who does it affect?	Trust	HA	PCG	PCT
2 *Continued*				
• Effective monitoring of clinical care with high-quality systems for clinical record keeping and the collection of relevant information.	✓		✓	✓
• Processes for assuring the quality of clinical care are in place and integrated with the quality programme for the organisation as a whole.	✓	✓	✓	✓
• Participation in well-designed, relevant R&D activity is encouraged and supported as something which can contribute to the development of an 'evaluation culture'.	✓	✓	✓	✓
3 Clear policies aimed at managing risks:				
• Controls assurance which promote self-assessment to identify and manage risks.	✓	✓	✓	✓
• Clinical risk systematically assessed with programmes in place to reduce risk.	✓			✓

Who does it affect?	Trust	HA	PCG	PCT
4 Procedures for all professional groups to identify and remedy poor performance, for example:				
• Critical incident reporting ensures that adverse events are identified, openly investigated, lessons are learned and promptly applied.	✓	✓	✓	✓
• Complaints procedures are accessible to patients and their families and fair to staff. Lessons are learned and recurrence of similar problems avoided.	✓	✓	✓	✓
• Professional performance procedures which take effect at an early stage before patients are harmed and which help the individual to improve their performance whenever possible, are in place and understood by all staff.	✓	✓	✓	✓
• Staff supported in their duty to report any concerns about colleagues' professional conduct and performance, with clear statements from the Board on what is expected of all staff. Clear procedures for reporting concerns so that early action can be taken to remedy the situation.	✓	✓	✓	✓

A check-up, from the neck up, to see if you've got your head around the essentials.

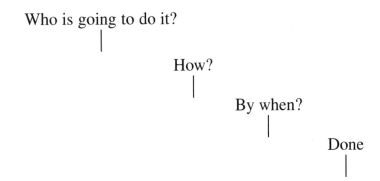

Who is going to do it?

How?

By when?

Done

1 Establish lead on CG.
2 Establish supporting committee.
3 Develop reporting systems for Board.
4 Baseline audit.
5 Action plan based on audit.
6 Review progress.
7 Quality process developed and integrated into organisation's processes.
8 Integrate targets for improvement into HImP.
9 Review working with organisations outside and across the NHS.
10 Improve working relationships with organisations above.
11 Systems for gathering best and evidence-based practice.
12 Systems for integrating improved practice into organisation.
13 Assessment of staff's continuing professional development needs.
14 Systems to support staff wishing to report concerns about conduct and performance of colleagues.
15 Risk analysis and response.
16 Liaison with patient and patient groups.
17 Material for annual CG report.
18 Review complaints procedures.
19 Systems to action remedies to adverse situations.
20 Identify poor clinical performance and take appropriate action.

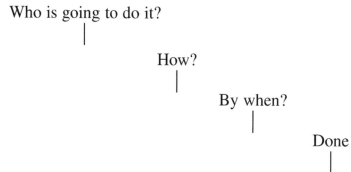

Who is going to do it?

How?

By when?

Done

21 Gather data and disseminate.
22 Monitor clinical care.
23 Consider action for visit from CHImP.

Now it's your turn – complete the list...

24
25
26
27
28
29

Start a new page if you need to!

Oh, just one more thing:

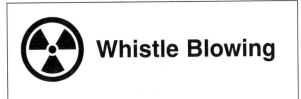

Whistle Blowing

Not a very nice phrase, but we know what it means. Recent events must have taught the NHS something about whistle blowing. Put another way, the ability of staff to highlight poor practice and performance without putting themselves or their career in jeopardy.

No one likes to be a 'grass' but who better to identify poor practice than the people on the ground doing the job. They know the difference between an honest mistake and an idiot, a trusted colleague and someone you wouldn't trust with a Barbie Doll. There is now a duty on staff to report any concerns they have about the conduct or performance of colleagues. The not unreasonable aim being to protect the best interests of the patients we serve and the organisations we work in.

CG creates the opportunity for a new understanding about whistle blowing and requires clear procedures for reporting concerns, so that early action can be taken to support the individual in order to remedy the situation.

Staff are to be supported in exercising their professional duty to report any concerns they may have about a colleague's fitness to practice, underlined by a clear statement from the CG Committee about what is expected of all staff.

Exercise

We all know the difficulties. Clinician and some management careers can depend on the patronage of senior colleagues and, later in life, the peers they trained with. Blowing the whistle is difficult enough. Sometimes it can be career terminating. Address the issue of confidentiality in whistle blowing. What system would you put in place to preserve, at least initially, the identity of a whistle blower and at the same time guard against frivolous or malicious complaints?

Exercise

What should be included in any statement about whistle blowing issued by the CG Committee?

The farmers and the cowmen must be friends

What happens when it looks like a doctor is going off the rails? I'm sure you know that *The farmers and the cowmen must be friends* is the title of a song from the hit musical *Oklahoma*. Or is it *Seven Brides for Seven Brothers*? I never can remember and no doubt you will tell me when you see me!

Anyway, it sort of describes the relationship there is/has been/should be between managers and medics. Managers and medics should be friends but often they are not. Few would deny that in large parts of the NHS there is a tension. There shouldn't be and there is no need for it, but there undeniably is.

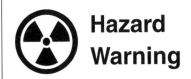

Hazard Warning

We should also have regard for the potential consequences for the doctor involved and consider the whole of the situation, with special regard to any underlying cause for poor performance.

Ways of detecting poor performance and practice early on are the best assurance that things don't get out of hand.

CG, with the pressure it is putting on all clinicians (not only medics) to improve their performance, has the potential to be an unwelcome pressure point. Reason? Well, although CG is a clinician-led initiative, it is managers who may well have to 'manage' the situation if things go wrong.

Particularly in secondary care, where it is a manager – the Trust Chief Executive – who is ultimately responsible for the clinical governance of his or her organisation, not a medic.

So, ways of detecting poor performance and practice early on are the best assurance that things don't get out of hand. Any procedures to support performance monitoring are probably best professionally-led – that way they're most likely to command the confidence of doctors.

Primarily, whatever we do as managers we must have the safety and peace of mind of patients as the goal. However, we should also have regard for the potential consequences for the doctor involved and consider the whole of the situation, with special regard to any underlying cause for poor performance.

How do you know when you've done it?

The idea is not to 'have done it'. CG is an ongoing process, certainly a 10-year roll out, as well as a process that commits itself to continuous improvement beyond that.

Central to CG is personal learning and continuous development – so CG is unrelenting! However, here are some questions that might provide the basis for benchmarking 'howyadoin' on the way.

 The questions are based on what colleagues in North Thames are doing, and a visit to their website via *http://www.doh.gov.uk/ntro/links.htm* would make a coffee break worthwhile.

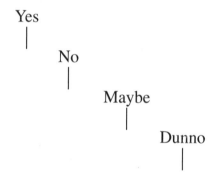

1 CG is accepted as integral to the management process?
2 CG is included in the business planning process and performance review?
3 CG involved clinicians in its formulation and achieved agreement about individual performance levels?
4 Local and regional performance levels are aligned (HA and PCGs are aligned)?
5 Staff accept the success criteria for measuring performance?
6 A few, meaningful, success criteria have been set? Such as:
   • organisational/cultural/environmental improvements
   • staff and organisational development
   • clinical audit
   • clinical risk management
   • clinical effectiveness.
7 Trusts have discussed CG objectives with region, and PCGs with HAs?
8 The Board are signed up to the objectives?

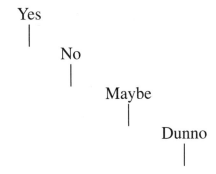

Yes

No

Maybe

Dunno

 9 The organisation is expressing its commitment
     to the development of staff by aiming for
     Investor in People Standards?

10 The Annual Report is a frank discussion of the
     organisation's CG position, and not a glossy
     make-over job? (Subjective but intuitive!)

11 Staff interviews record improvements in
     attitude and perceptions about CG?

12 All professional staff have personal
     development plans?

13 Staff receive on going education and training
     relevant to their clinical practice?

14 Clinical directors have job descriptions
     describing responsibilities for clinical
     quality and what to do about poorly
     performing staff and have received
     appropriate training?

15 Action plans, built on baseline evaluations, are
     reviewed each year and outcomes audited?

16 Where audits are used to review standards,
     explicit improvement criteria are set?

17 Move towards involving more staff and
     departments in CG audit activity? Specific
     targets are set for widening involvement with
     the aim of involving all staff by an agreed
     date?

18 Regular development of multi-disciplinary,
     multi-Trust, multi-sectoral team working?

19 Widen audit to include multi-disciplinary,
     multi-Trust, multi-sectoral activity with targets
     to widen the groups included?

20 Evaluation to determine changes to patient
     care?

21 Adoption of policies to encourage a blame
     free, open, learning culture?

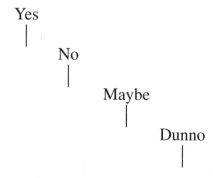

22 Risk management systems are in place throughout the organisation with regular updates and reports?

23 A process of managing complaints and claims that minimises stress to patients and staff in place?

24 Benefits to patient care are identified as a result of action following complaints investigation?

25 Regular meetings with patient groups and surveys show demonstrable improvements?

26 Dissemination of effectiveness bulletins and similar?

27 NICE guidelines are implemented with action plan for non-compliance as routine? Audit for compliance?

28 CG Committee examines national guidelines and protocols and checks against local performance?

29 Development of clinical pathways across all clinical directorates?

30 Your place is a happy, safe and interesting place to work?

Is there anyone else doing all the CG stuff?

Fear not, you are not alone!

Here are some websites you might like to visit to find out more about CG and how other people are dealing with it.

What, not wired? Go and polish your gas lamp!

Time for a coffee and a browse around the wonderful world of cyberspace. Try the following:

http://www.doh.gov.uk/nyro/clingov/cghome.htm

http://www.doh.gov.uk/pricare/index.htm

http://www.shef.ac.uk/uni/projects/wrp/cgconf.html

http://www.bamm.co.uk/clinical.htm

http://www.doh.gov.uk/ntro/summary.htm

http://www.xnet.com/~hret/weine324.htm

http://www.cyberscape.co.uk/bvhaps/bpclinef.htm

http://www.nzgg.org.nz/

http://www.cyberscape.co.uk/bvhaps/!clineff.htm

http://www.pcs.mgh.harvard.edu/

http://www.rcgp.org.uk/courses/

There are many other interesting international health listings to be found at www.roylilley.co.uk

Did you come up with anything interesting? The sites change all the time as does their content. If you find a really, really good one let me know, please! Just try searching under 'clinical governance' and see what you come up with.